8-19-05

Nancy L. Beckerman, LCSW, DSW

Couples of Mixed HIV Status
Clinical Issues and Interventions

Pre-publication REVIEWS, COMMENTARIES, EVALUATIONS . . .

"**D**r. Beckerman has provided therapists with a greatly needed tool to assist in the counseling of couples of mixed HIV status. Her current research and application of theoretical models provides important guidance in addressing issues of high prevalence among these couples. Especially valuable is her consideration of these issues across the variables of race, gender, and sexual orientation. For many years those of us working in human services with HIV-positive persons have talked about 'living with AIDS'; in this book Dr. Beckerman provides clinicians with the tools to address this central issue in the emotional lives of persons living with AIDS and those whom they love and who love them."

Jay Laudato, LMSW
Executive Director,
Callen-Lorde Community Health Center

"**T**his book is a gold mine for the mental health clinician working with couples of mixed HIV status. The author has carefully researched recurring psychosocial challenges in a sizable sample of couples of mixed status (both gay and straight) and has identified a set of key challengers that are of most concern to these couples. For partners who are negotiating the many complex emotional, medical, and sexual challenges of being a couple of mixed HIV status, the author describes quite clearly several intervention frameworks for couples' therapy, then guides us as to which framework works best, under what circumstances, and why.

The many rich clinical vignettes and session transcripts bring clients' concerns to life and help the clinician more fully understand how to best use one's 'therapeutic self.' A winner!"

Vincent J. Lynch, PhD, MSW
Founder and Chair,
The Annual National Conference
on Social Work and HIV/AIDS;
Director of Continuing Education
and Adjunct Associate Professor,
Boston College Graduate School
of Social Work

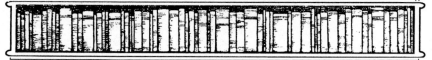

More pre-publication
REVIEWS, COMMENTARIES, EVALUATIONS . . .

"Incandescent, intelligent, and informative. Nancy L. Beckerman offers an insightful and well-researched look at the intimate lives of the sero-discordant couple. The gentle candor in her writing demonstrates practicality and compassion in response to the new realities of HIV-positive people and those who treat them. Particular strengths are evident when she invites us into her therapy sessions, guiding not only her patients but us as clinicians as well. It is at the intersection of HIV and couples' therapy where the author shines with both clarity and confidence."

Michael Mancilla, MSW, LICSW
Co-Author, *Love in the Time of HIV:*
The Gay Man's Guide to Sex, Dating,
and Relationships

The Haworth Press®
New York • London • Oxford

Couples of Mixed HIV Status
Clinical Issues and Interventions

Haworth Psychosocial Issues of HIV/AIDS
R. Dennis Shelby, PhD
Senior Editor

HIV and Social Work: A Practitioner's Guide edited by David M. Aronstein and Bruce J. Thompson

HIV/AIDS and the Drug Culture: Shattered Lives by Elizabeth Hagan and Joan Gormley

AIDS and Mental Health Practice: Clinical and Policy Issues edited by Michael Shernoff

AIDS and Development in Africa: A Social Science Perspective by Kempe Ronald Hope Sr.

Women's Experiences with HIV/AIDS: Mending Fractured Selves by Desirée Ciambrone

Hotel Ritz—Comparing Mexican and U.S. Street Prostitutes: Factors in HIV/AIDS Transmission by David J. Bellis

Practice Issues in HIV/AIDS Services: Empowerment-Based Models and Program Applications edited by Ronald J. Mancoske and James Donald Smith

Preventing AIDS: Community-Science Collaborations edited by Benjamin P. Bowser, Shiraz I. Mishra, Cathy J. Reback, and George F. Lemp

Couples of Mixed HIV Status: Clinical Issues and Interventions by Nancy L. Beckerman

Lesbian Women and Sexual Health: The Social Construction of Risk and Susceptibility by Kathleen A. Dolan

Behind the Eight Ball: Sex for Crack Cocaine Exchange and Poor Black Women by Tanya Telfair Sharpe

Couples of Mixed HIV Status
Clinical Issues and Interventions

Nancy L. Beckerman, LCSW, DSW

The Haworth Press®
New York • London • Oxford

For more information on this book or to order, visit
http://www.haworthpress.com/store/product.asp?sku=5327

or call 1-800-HAWORTH (800-429-6784) in the United States and Canada
or (607) 722-5857 outside the United States and Canada

or contact orders@HaworthPress.com

PUBLISHER'S NOTE
Identities and circumstances of individuals discussed in this book have been changed to protect
confidentiality.

The Haworth Press, Inc., 10 Alice Street, Binghamton, NY 13904-1580.

Cover design by Lora Wiggins.

Library of Congress Cataloging-in-Publication Data

Beckerman, Nancy L.
    Couples of mixed HIV status : clinical issues and interventions / Nancy L. Beckerman.
        p. ; cm.
    Includes bibliographical references and index.
    ISBN 0-7890-1851-9 (hard : alk. paper) — ISBN 0-7890-1852-7 (soft : alk. paper)
    1. HIV-positive persons. 2. Couples. 3. Marital psychotherapy. [DNLM: 1. HIV Infections—
psychology. 2. Couples Therapy—methods. 3. HIV Infections—prevention & control. WC 503.7
B396c 2005] I. Title.

RC606.6.B44 2005
362.196'9792—dc22
                                                                                    2004027746

CONTENTS

ABOUT THE AUTHOR

Nancy L. Beckerman, LCSW, DSW, is an associate professor at Wurzweiler School of Social Work, Yeshiva University in New York. In her private practice, she provides clinical services to the HIV/AIDS community. She is a consultant and supervisor, specializing in couple and family therapy. Dr. Beckerman has published extensively on HIV/AIDS, couple and family therapy, and health and mental health in social work. Her research, practice, and supervisions center around couple therapy and in particular, the psychological impact of chronic illness on couples' relationships.

Prologue

RATIONALE

In my experience as a clinician providing couple therapy to numerous couples affected by HIV, certain issues repeatedly emerged in therapy that were both universal and unique to couples of mixed HIV status. The psychosocial impact of illness may pose intrapsychic and dyadic challenges, such as coping with uncertainty and the shifting of emotional and functional roles, regardless of the nature of the medical illness. When turning to relevant literature and research to help refine techniques with this population, I found that the literature largely reflected the era prior to combination therapies, identifying relationship issues such as loss and bereavement and caregiving. My clinical experience suggested that the relevant literature lacked discussion about the types of dyadic emotional challenges that were emerging in clinical practice and the theoretical frameworks that could be applied effectively. Issues such as fear of HIV transmission between partners, disclosure of HIV status to each other and to others, issues of mistrust and betrayal provoked by the HIV diagnosis, and the impact of an HIV diagnosis on family planning could be further studied and clarified for clinicians providing services to this population.

A research study of forty-four serodiscordant couples in the Northeast served as a starting point for this inquiry of distinctive relationship issues confronting couples of mixed HIV status. This book provides an overview of the findings from this research, as well as an application of those couple-therapy approaches that have proved particularly effective in the treatment of couples of mixed HIV status. Based on this research and extensive case studies, this book provides an introduction for therapists who are interested in (1) understanding the unique emotional challenges of couples of mixed HIV status, and (2) gaining a theoretical base that can inform their practice with couples of mixed HIV status. Information about what couples may experience and relevant theoretical applications can be used by any marriage or family therapist to guide the nature of their interventions with this population. This book will also be helpful to the student of counseling and health-related services, as well as the lay reader who may be in a serodiscordant relationship, or the friends or family members of couples living with HIV.

PLAN OF THE BOOK

This book is organized to introduce the therapist to the unique emotional challenges that may face couples of mixed HIV status and provide a range of theoretical approaches that can be employed effectively. The historical context of HIV/AIDS and couples of mixed HIV status and relevant literature are provided as a foundation in Chapters 1 and 2. Chapter 3 includes the historical and current overview of couple therapy frameworks that are of particular relevance to therapists counseling couples of mixed HIV status. The central frameworks of emotionally focused couple therapy (EFCT), integrative couple therapy (ICT), medical family therapy, and structural couple therapy are discussed in detail and other relevant approaches are also reviewed. The reader is then introduced to the research methodology and findings in Chapters 4 and 5. Chapters 6 through 11 are each devoted to one of the six issues commonly identified. Each chapter identifies and analyzes the findings, both empirical and qualitative. After identifying each issue in each chapter, case studies are used to further illustrate how these issues may manifest themselves differently with diverse couples and how theoretical frameworks can be applied differentially depending on different issues and varied sociocultural and characterological factors. The case studies are used to demonstrate how these variables may be addressed in the dynamic context of the clinical realm. In the epilogue, the conclusion provides a summary of key findings and implications for the therapist providing couple therapy to couples of mixed HIV status. This book can be used as a resource for therapists working with today's couples of mixed HIV status.

Chapter 1

Introduction

Disease may destroy only a few cells or an entire organism, and with it, the individual. For this reason, man suffers and is afraid: disease reminds him that he is mortal . . . that he is alone and must die sooner or later. Elementary fears . . . come from the depth of the unconscious, breaking through the thin crust of security.

H. E. Sigerist (1943, p. 6)

The crisis of physical illness comes to each individual and each couple in ways both universal and unique. When one partner in a relationship has been diagnosed with HIV, the couple may experience a unique tier of relationship conflicts above and beyond what any couple facing another physical illness may experience.* Because of the populations affected, unpredictable treatment, stigma, and transmissibility, couples of mixed HIV status must contend with a range of emotional reactions both individually and as a dyad. The distinct nature of HIV/AIDS creates conflicts and intensifies preexisting conflicts in the relationship in its own unique way.

Based on a research study (forty-four couples) with couples of mixed HIV status,** this book provides an identification and analysis of the types of relationship issues that commonly arise for serodiscordant couples. Some of these issues are universal, such as shifts in

---

*The term *HIV* throughout the book will refer to asymptomatic HIV. When *HIV/AIDS* is used, it will refer to disease progression marked by HIV-related illness.

**The term *couples of mixed HIV status* will refer to couples in which one partner has tested HIV positive and one partner has tested HIV negative. At times, relevant literature refers to this phenomenon as *serodiscordant couples.*

emotional intimacy due to the diagnosis and coping with uncertainty, and some are particular to what a couple of mixed HIV status might contend with, such as fear of HIV transmission between partners, disclosing a partner's status, feelings of betrayal, and family planning issues. The analysis of these HIV/AIDS issues in couples as demographics and treatments continues to evolve.

The focus of this book is on identifying and clarifying the unique emotional issues common to couples of mixed HIV status. Once presented, assessment and intervention are discussed from several couple-therapy frameworks, primarily that of emotionally focused couple therapy (EFCT) and integrative couple therapy (ICT). These and other couple-therapy frameworks are reviewed and illustrated in their application to several couples in practice. In this way, practitioners can conceptualize how they might employ practice principles with both the universal and unique emotional challenges couples of mixed HIV status may face.

KEY EMOTIONAL ISSUES

The dyadic issues of couples of mixed HIV status often are superimposed on issues or conflicts that predate the HIV diagnosis, maybe even predate this particular relationship. Multifaceted variables such as characterological tendencies and illness in family of origin must be considered, as well as the impact of illness issues experienced by the individual and his or her partner in the face of a potentially life-altering illness.

As any medical social worker knows, psychosocial issues such as coping and adaptation, denial and acceptance, independence and dependence, and hope and despair are at the vortex of emotional reactions to illness affecting not only the individual, but the couple and family as well (Baider and Sarrell, 1984; Baider and Spexiele, 1997; Campbell and Patterson, 1995; Frazier, Davis-Ali, and Dahl, 1995; Gotay, 1984; Krausz, 1988; Lyons, 1995; McDaniel, Hepworth, and Doherty, 1995; Moos and Tzu, 1977; Parker, 1993; Rolland, 1994; Sabo, Brown, and Smith, 1986; Spexiele, 1997). Although broad conceptual frameworks may have informed social work practitioners through such reactions, specific sensitive challenges exist that singularly affect couples of mixed HIV status. These issues may include: how and when one partner contracted HIV, issues of mistrust or betrayal, fear of HIV transmission within the relationship, stigma, and disclosure issues. Family planning dilemmas have emerged in the more recent literature on couples of mixed HIV status (Avert, 2002; Beckerman, Letteney, and Lorber, 2001; Katz, 1997; Leask et al., 1997; Klitzman, 1997; MacDonald, 1998; Pasquier et al., 2000; Scarce, 1999; Williams-Saporito, 1998).

Through the 1980s and 1990s, couples of mixed HIV status have had to cope primarily with issues surrounding physical and psychological impacts of illness, loss, caregiving strains, impact of stigma, mourning, and bereavement (Burgoyne, 1994; Christ and Wiener, 1984; Foley et al., 1994; Folkman, Chesney, and Christopher-Richards, 1994; Geis, Fuller, and Rush, 1986; Lippmann, James, and Frierson, 1993; Pearlin, Semple, and Turner, 1993; Powell-Cope, 1995; Rowe, Plum, and Crossman, 1988; Shelby, 1992; Stulberg and Buckingham, 1988).

There has been only limited discussion of family systems and self-psychology as effective approaches with the intrapsychic and interpersonal issues in the realm of HIV/AIDS (Walker, 1991; Shelby, 1992). Social workers have counseled their clients through the developmental cycle starting with the crisis of HIV testing, and moving through numerous health crises until sadly reaching grief and bereavement after the loss of a partner (Buckingham, 1987; Burgoyne, 1994; Folkman, Chesney, and Christoper-Richards, 1994; Powell-Cope, 1996). HIV/AIDS social workers and other mental health practitioners who counsel couples coping with HIV in their lives have applied systemic and psychotherapeutic approaches, but relied predominantly on a psychosocial model based on principles such as coping and adaptation to illness and loss from crisis intervention and bereavement approaches (Bor, Miller, and Goldman 1993; Grace, 1994; Hoffman, 1991; Rait, Ross, and Rao, 1997; Shelby, 1995; Winiarski, 1991).

The knowledge base and practice skills adapted from crisis intervention and bereavement provided effective conceptual frameworks for practitioners for the first 20 years of HIV/AIDS. However, given the compelling advances in HIV/AIDS treatments that have consistently lowered AIDS deaths since 1997 (CDC, 1998, 1999, 2000,

2001), crisis and bereavement frameworks may no longer be the exclusive or most effective framework for counseling couples of mixed HIV status. For those who have responded well to new combination therapies, many are returning to life-affirming activities and relationships. Those already in long-term relationships are more able to shift their emotional energy away from illness and dying, and more toward maintaining and enhancing their primary relationships (Anderson and Weatherburn, 1998; Beckerman, Letteney, and Lorber, 2001; Greenan and Tunnell, 2003; Mancilla and Troshinsky, 2003; Mayer and Wells, 1997; Moore et al., 1998; Pomeroy, Green, and Van Laningham, 2002; Powell-Cope, 1996; Remien, 1998; VanDevanter, Clearly, and Moore, 1998; Van der Straten et al., 1998). Theoretical approaches, such as medical family therapy, emotionally focused couple therapy (EFCT), and integrative couple therapy (ICT), that have been particularly effective with these issues are introduced and illustrated through each chapter and each case study.

INTRODUCTION TO RESEARCH STUDY

The identification of emotional issues common to couples of mixed HIV status is based on findings from an exploratory research study of forty-four couples of mixed HIV status, as well as the clinical immersion (numerous cases) of therapeutic contact. Six primary issues are identified. Respondents from the study were asked to answer open-ended questions, and their narrative responses are provided to further illustrate the types of emotional issues that have been consistently identified by couples of mixed HIV status. Couples who have been treated, duly disguised, are presented through case studies to provide further depth and context of how ongoing relationships are affected when one partner is HIV positive. These trends and case studies are shared and analyzed to assist practitioners in refining their conceptual framework and skill base for practice with couples of mixed HIV status.

HOW THIS BOOK IS ORGANIZED

Chapter 2 provides a historical context of HIV and couples, and reviews the empirical and nonempirical research and literature on the topic. In Chapter 3, selected theoretical orientations within couple therapy are reviewed to provide a more responsive treatment approach to some of the common issues couples of mixed HIV status may present. The methodology of the study, including the design, data collection, the instrument, and data analysis are provided in Chapter 4. The identification and explanation of the results are introduced in Chapter 5 and analysis and discussion of the six commonly identified emotional issues are found in Chapters 6 through 11. Salient clinical issues are analyzed to provide illumination for couples and potential guidelines for practitioners at the end of each of these chapters. The epilogue provides a summary of clinical issues and interventions for conjoint therapy with couples of mixed HIV status.

For those providing individual and couple counseling around HIV issues, the book will provide information and insight into a broader conceptual framework of the issues that are likely to present with couples of mixed HIV status, and theoretical orientations within couple therapy that can be used effectively when treating serodiscordant couples. This book can be used for any individual or couple affected by HIV/AIDS, as well as family members, parents, siblings, and friends of any couple affected by HIV/AIDS who may wish to better understand and cope with their emotional experiences surrounding HIV in their lives.

Chapter 2

Literature Review

HISTORICAL CONTEXT OF HIV/AIDS AND COUPLES

To appreciate how couples of mixed HIV status are affected by HIV in their lives, one needs to understand the potent historical context of HIV/AIDS in the United States. The heady air of gay sexual liberation of the 1970s is now understood as the ironic prologue to 1979, the year that marked the very first mysterious moments of a serious set of maladies affecting young men. Symptoms such as dermatological rashes and lesions, a rare form of unusually potent pneumonia, and enlarged lymph nodes puzzled and stumped the first set of physicians exposed to this phenomena (CDC, 1981; Curran, 1983). Within months, this handful of physicians on both coasts of the United States noted another trend in their respective patients: they were all gay men. As Greenan and Tunnell (2003) explain, the uprising of the gay community at the Stonewall Inn in 1969 brought being gay into the public spotlight, but AIDS brought gay male couples to the forefront of media attention.

The first article on HIV that appeared in the mainstream press *(The New York Times)* was printed in 1981: "Rare Cancer Seen in 41 Homosexuals" (Mass, 1987). This "rare cancer" appeared to be deadly. Those studying this phenomenon assumed it had something to with the gay social behaviors of its recipients and dubbed it gay related immune disorder or GRID (Curran, 1983). GRID received startlingly little coverage in the first few years: seven articles in *The New York Times* over eighteen months when the number of reported AIDS cases went from forty-one to 1,200. This was experienced as a direct message by some in the gay community that their deaths were unimportant and perhaps, wanted by some outside of the gay community (Kramer, 1989).

Those living and dying with GRID or the "gay plague," as it was referred to inside and outside of the gay community, had little or no information about an illness that struck swiftly and decidedly and appeared to be working its way through circles of friends (Curran, 1983; Dowdle, 1983). GRID, and then in 1983, under the new name of acquired immune deficiency syndrome (AIDS) challenged mainstream society to confront mortality in an era that was becoming accustomed to almost routinely conquering death with the use of life-sustaining treatments, such as respirators, dialysis, and transplantation.

Individuals living with AIDS were flooded by feelings of fear and terror. There were no explanations of the origin or any possible treatments for this swift, disfiguring terminal illness. In addition to intense fear, those affected by AIDS experienced intense stigma by friends and family. Even those in the health care system and many communities across the country saw the disease as gay related. Intense stigma resulted in repeated scenarios of violence and discrimination toward those diagnosed with AIDS (Bacon, 1987; Christ and Wiener, 1986; Hausman, 1983; Kaisch and Anton-Culver, 1989). In some circumstances even those related to the identified patient were victimized with acts of hate and violence (Bacon, 1987; Martin, 1989; McKusick, Horstman, and Carfagni, 1983). Many people living with AIDS withdrew and chose not to disclose their health status (Hausman, 1983). The partners of those living with AIDS experienced intense trepidation about the disease progression and impending loss, as well as feelings of despair and isolation in the face of the widespread stigma associated with the disease (Christ and Wiener, 1986; Rowe, Plum, and Crossman, 1988; Stulberg and Buckingham, 1988).

Through the mid-1980s, the demographic face of HIV/AIDS shifted to include spiraling rates of HIV-infected women. In the United States, cumulative demographics of HIV-infected gay men (or in CDC terminology, men who have sex with men) totaled 368,971, and the number of women who were exposed through heterosexual contact was up to 57,396 from 7 percent of overall HIV population in 1985 to 26 percent in 1993 (CDC, 2001). The medical community, public health structures, and mainstream media began to understand this was no longer a "gay plague" but an indiscriminate, transmissible virus that seriously, even fatally impaired one's immune system. Heterosexual couples with women almost exclusively of childbearing age and their male partners became a growing focus of media attention.

During the 1980s, community-based organizations, AIDS service organizations, and hospitals serving people with AIDS still largely conceptualized HIV/AIDS as an individual plight. Support groups were separately provided for people with AIDS (PWAs) and care partners respectively. The gay male culture still emphasized individual autonomy and was not typically welcoming to couples coping with HIV/AIDS. The larger heterosexist culture still has not affirmed gay male couples, not offering legal or religious sanctions or financial benefits. This has to be understood as a historical and current component in the range of psychosocial conflicts in serodiscordant relationships among gay males. Although the mainstream media, largely television and film entertainment, has shifted in many superficial ways to include the gay community, even profitted from it in the television market (*Will & Grace, Queer Eye for the Straight Guy*, etc.), much of what is now accepted is still wildly stereotypical and does not signify a fundamental inclusion marked by social, religious, and legal measures that provide equity with the heterosexual community.

Another component in the lives of serodiscordant couples is the changing treatment of HIV/AIDS over the years and how it affects the individual and dyadic functioning of the couple. With the introduction of AZT in 1987, the mortality rates of those living with HIV/AIDS improved significantly for a short period (CDC, 1989; CDC, 1990). Couples still were challenged by emotional reactions to diagnosis, fear of HIV transmission within the relationship, issues surrounding disclosure and caregiving, and were now faced with new and different emotional challenges regarding medication (Broder, 1989; Mancilla and Troshinsky, 2003; Mayer and Wells, 1997; Pearlin, Semple, and Turner, 1993; Strug, Grube, and Beckerman, 2002). These included adherence to often complicated medication regimes and the impact of how these regimes often intruded on a sense of normalcy. In many circumstances, intensely uncomfortable side effects caused more complications than disease progression. Fear often loomed for the serodiscordant couples that the medications would be intolerable, or if tolerated, abruptly diminish in ability to keep one's viral load low. Couples continued to struggle with persistent and painful levels of uncertainty about their futures.

As HIV/AIDS treatments advanced with the introduction of protease inhibitors in combination with reverse transcriptase inhibitors (highly active antiretroviral therapy or HAART) in 1996, AIDS mortality rates were significantly reduced (CDC, 2001; Swanstrom and Erona, 2000; Vitinghoff et al., 1999). There have been ever-changing combinations of antiretroviral drug regimens, each with different success rates of lowering viral loads and decreasing HIV-resistant mutations. For those who have had access to these treatments and have been able to tolerate a range of potent side effects, the quality and length of life has been improved. Those responding well have shifted from anticipating death to trying to live with HIV/AIDS with guarded optimism (Beckerman, Letteney, and Lorber, 2001; Mancilla and Troshinsky, 2003; Remien, 1998).

It is important to note that there has been an increase in HIV-associated illnesses, such as hepatitis C. Hepatitis C is a liver disease caused by the hepatitis C virus (HCV), which is spread by contact with the blood of an HCV-infected person. The virus can remain dormant in the liver system until it is triggered by a range of behavioral activities, such as alcoholism, drug overdose, or a depleted immune system. In fact, researchers and medical practitioners who specialize in liver disease and HIV/AIDS suggest that HCV should be seen as an opportunistic infection (Dietrich, 2001). Nationally, an estimated 33 to 40 percent of people with HIV/AIDS are also infected with HCV, and HCV has become one of the leading causes of death among persons with HIV/AIDS (Carruthers et al., 2001). Typical symptoms of HCV include jaundice, acute fatigue, abdominal pain, loss of appetite, and nausea. It can be life threatening if an individual cannot tolerate the juggling of medication regimes. This represents an additional significant biopsychosocial challenge for those living with both disease processes (Carruthers et al., 2001).

Nevertheless, there continues to be optimism about the overall improvement found in combination therapies since the mid-1990s. With more effective treatment advances, long-term HIV survivors are turning their attention back toward career and relationship challenges (Grube, Beckerman, and Strug, 2003; Remien, 1998; Powell-Cope, 1995). Recent research on couples of mixed HIV status is provided with an overview of the empirical studies and their outcomes as well as relevant anecdotal reports from literature.

EMPIRICAL RESEARCH
ON SERODISCORDANT COUPLES

In 2002, Pomeroy, Green, and Van Laningham examined the effectiveness of a psychoeducational group intervention for serodiscordant heterosexual couples.

Although this was a small study (several groups of serodiscordant couples), the authors found that group intervention was an effective venue for reducing depression and anxiety that results from HIV in serodiscordant heterosexual couples.

Palmer and Bor (2001) facilitated a multiple case study of ten serodiscordant gay male couples residing in London to develop a better understanding of the unique psychosocial tasks often confronting couples of mixed HIV status. Semistructured interviews were held with general lines of inquiry including the impact of such issues as disclosure of diagnosis, availability and provision of emotional support, impact of diagnosis on the sexual relationship, and the future of the relationship. After case analysis, the authors found that the presence of HIV and potential future illness "create an imbalance in long-term HIV-serodiscordant gay male relationships" (Palmer and Bor, 2001, p. 1). Specifically, this imbalance emerged in unsettling patterns of sexual and emotional intimacy. Although couples reported a range of consequences to their sexual lives together, with several reporting no sexual activity since diagnosis, most noteworthy were the two out of ten couples in which the seronegative partner intentionally tried to contract HIV in order to address the imbalance in the relationship. This is an important finding as it is not as unusual as one might think, and should be further researched and examined. Regarding the emotional challenges facing couples, the authors highlight the strain of the HIV-negative partner being in the "caretaker" role. Being put into this role, and accepting it, contributes to relationship tensions, inequities, and perhaps emotional distancing. The authors report that the HIV-negative partner is more likely to be the caregiver and therefore may hold more emotional and practical power. Overall, the key finding then was the prevalence of relationship imbalance due to the difference in serostatus.

Beckerman, Letteney, and Lorber (2001) explored the emotional challenges and conflicts commonly experienced by individuals in a serodiscordant relationship (n = 82). The participants represented heterosexual and gay partnerships almost equally. Individuals were surveyed using a 25-item scale developed for the study which sought to identify existing issues and their relative frequencies. Several open-ended questions were used to capture nuances that may have been missed by the Likert-scale format. The authors found six key issues that were identified by at least half of the sample. In order of high conflict to moderate conflict, they are:

1. fear of HIV transmission,
2. coping with uncertainty,
3. shifts in emotional intimacy,
4. impact on sexuality,
5. disclosure issues, and
6. dilemmas regarding reproductive choices (Beckerman, Letteney, and Lorber, 2001).

VanDevanter and colleagues (1999) explored unique psychosocial issues confronting serodiscordant couples by using qualitative data from sixty support groups for HIV-discordant couples. Over a two-year period from 1992-1994, data from forty-one couples who had participated in voluntary support groups were analyzed by content analysis with an aim toward identifying psychosocial challenges and issues. Four primary issues emerged as common to the majority of serodiscordant couples: (1) dealing with the emotional and sexual impact on their relationship; (2) confronting reproductive decisions; (3) planning for the future of children and the surviving partner, and (4) disclosure of the HIV infection to friends and family.

Van der Straten and colleagues (1998) conducted a qualitative study based on a small convenience sample (n = 28) out of a larger ongoing study (Van der Straten et al., 1998). The study participants were partners in HIV-discordant relationships and were interviewed regarding the role of serostatus and stigma in shaping their emotional experiences surrounding HIV, sex, and risk. Key findings included the identification of the common dynamic that the difference in serostatus often created feelings of emotional distance and alienation within the relationship, as well as the feeling of being segregated by the health care community according to serostatus. In addition, sero-discordant couples identified ongoing conflict around issues of disclosure, and difficulty negotiating emotional feelings regarding their sexual relationship. These issues were addressed most effectively by access to HIV information and to other serodiscordant couples (Van der Straten et al., 1998).

Klitzman (1997), based on interviews with thirty-eight HIV-positive men and women, provides a narrative of the unique and common experiences of being HIV positive. Klitzman's work gives voice to how HIV-positive individuals experience the common emotional challenges related to HIV.

Adam and Sears (1996) interviewed sixty HIV-positive individuals and forty caregivers (those caring for the HIV-infected individual, not necessarily partners). The sample consisted of both gay (n = 41) and heterosexual (n = 7) men and women in southwestern Ontario and southeastern Michigan. The study found that negotiating safer sex was of utmost concern for both partners in couples of mixed HIV status. Fear of infecting one's HIV-negative partner was of equal concern as the fear of being infected by one's partner.

Remien, Carballo-Dieguez, and Wagner (1995) reported preliminary findings based on fifteen serodiscordant gay male couples in New York. Many factors related to how HIV affected the couples' sexual relationship were identified; age, ethnicity, length of relationship, established behavioral patterns, levels of sexual and emotional intimacy, and substance abuse. Couples consistently identified uncertainty as a key emotional challenge. The range of uncertainty varied and included feelings of uncertainty in relation to the course of the disease, uncertainty about transmitting the virus, and uncertainty about caregiving concerns (Remien, 1998). An insidious apprehension was described by couples as soon as a positive test result was received and this apprehension continued throughout their years together (Folkman, Chesney, and Christopher-Richards, 1994; Shelby, 1992).

Powell-Cope (1995) reported on five serodiscordant couples and found an anxious uncertainty looming. This uncertainty largely involved the arrival of acute illness and how each partner might respond to a serious AIDS-related illness, e.g., with fear, withdrawal, or dependency (Powell-Cope, 1995).

Foley and colleagues (1994) conducted a study to determine the extent to which family members of couples of mixed HIV status were aware of the HIV-positive status of their family member, and to what extent they were perceived as supportive to the serodiscordant couple. From 1990 to 1992, 109 serodiscordant couples were interviewed. The key findings included: (1) the higher the education of the couples of mixed HIV status, the less likely they were to disclose to families of origin, (2) Fewer HIV-negative partners had family members aware (only 50 percent informed their families) than HIV-positive partners (75 percent) who largely experienced more support, (3) those who were African American had the lowest levels of disclosure to their families of origin, and (4) mothers and sisters were perceived as significantly more supportive to the couple than fathers and brothers.

A body of anecdotal work has also emerged that provides an overview of the psychosocial impact for partners caring for loved ones with HIV/AIDS since the late 1980s. Relevant literature from the early era of HIV/AIDS identified some of the challenges facing couples of mixed HIV status, such as shock, denial, anticipatory grief, fear of HIV transmission, multiple losses, issues of disclosing one's HIV status to both families, shifts in emotional intimacy, and intense stigma (Burgoyne, 1994; Gels, Fuller, and Rush, 1986; Hoffman, 1991; Klimes et al., 1992; Stulberg and Buckingham, 1988; Weitz, 1989).

Most of this literature was written prior to the advent of combination therapy, and there is also a decided emphasis on how caregiving strains affect the relationship (Bor, Miller, and Goldman, 1993; Folkman, Chesney, and Christopher-Richards, 1994; Lippmann, James, and Frierson, 1993; Powell-Cope and Brown, 1992).

The phases that Shelby (1992) developed as a conceptual framework were particularly responsive to the range of intrapsychic and interpersonal issues that accompanies a couple from the anxiety of HIV diagnosis, through disease progression, to the sad denouement of bereavement with the occurrence of untimely death of one partner. Still of direct relevance for understanding what serodiscordant couples go through is the couple's ongoing emotional conflicts as they try to negotiate the challenges of simultaneously balancing fear of illness with wishes for life-affirming intimacy.

More recently, anecdotal literature supports the presence of already identified psychosocial challenges such as coping with uncertainty, fear of HIV transmission, potential caregiving strains, disclosure, and issues of stigma (Leask et al., 1997; Moore et al., 1998). Emerging literature identifies how combination therapies have affected the lives of couples of mixed HIV status, and points to the tensions surrounding medication adherence, fear that positive benefits will not last, and of course the many challenges of coping with side effects (Anderson and Weatherburn, 1998).

Mancilla and Troshinsky (2003) provide the first comprehensive handbook for living and coping with HIV/AIDS directed toward gay men. Important issues are identified and guidance is offered to individuals and couples living with HIV in their relationships. Essentially, Mancilla and Troshinsky (2003) provide psychosocial skills and tools for coping with the effects that HIV may have on individuals and partners in their dating or established relationships. Guidelines are outlined for such common challenges as disclosing one's HIV status to a partner, (who to tell, when to tell, how to tell), how to keep love and sex vibrant between HIV-positive partners and serodiscordant partners, how to keep sex as safe as possible between partners, and how to sustain mutual trust and equity between gay male partners.

In established serodiscordant relationships, there are unique complexities in the emotional and sexual dynamics that are identified and explored (Mancilla and Troshinsky, 2003; Beckerman, Letteney, and Lorber, 2001). Fear of HIV transmission continues to persist, but may be somewhat lower than before high active antiretroviral therapies became available (Beckerman, Letteney, and Lorber, 2001). However it is not uncommon that the serodiscordant couple experiences a diminution of a satisfying sex life. This may be temporary and may be due to a variety of biological factors, such as lower testosterone levels, disease progression, or side effects from medication. It also not uncommon that the anxiety and depression that accompany an HIV diagnosis or an HIV-related illness may rob one or both partners of a sexual appetite (Mancilla and Troshinsky, 2003).

Other current issues include adherence to combination therapy regimes, side effects of these therapies, and development of preemptive therapies, such as postexposure prophylaxis (PEP), which is provided to health care workers after exposure to HIV to interrupt progression to infection. If such preemptive therapies become widely available, this may be of particular relevance to serodiscordant couples. With more effective medications, serodiscordant couples are still experiencing emotional reactions to living with the uncertainty of their HIV diagnosis. Uncertainty about disease progression very often continues to consume both partners, and emotional responses include gearing up and rushing toward intimacy (because time suddenly seems short) or being rendered unable to move forward by depression and pessimistic thoughts (Mancilla and Troshinsky, 2003).

As always, issues of caretaking exist even with an asymptomatic partner; many HIV-negative partners feel overprotective and institute dynamics in which they make more and more decisions that should be mutual (Greenan and Tunnell, 2003; Mancilla and Troshinsky, 2003). Another issue regarding serodiscordant couples that has recently emerged and appears to primarily impact heterosexual couples is how HIV affects the decisions regarding reproduction and parenthood (Avert, 2002; Beckerman, Beder, and Gelman, 1996; Kalichman and Nachimson, 1999; Pasquier et al., 2000). Emotional and ethical dilemmas exist for couples who want to have children but are conflicted about the potential harm to the woman who may be HIV negative, or to the fetus that may be infected by an HIV-positive mother (Beckerman, Beder, and Gelman, 1996; Beckerman and Gelman, 2000). As advanced medication treatments such as antiretroviral drugs have decreased perinatal transmission to nearly 2 to 3 percent, more HIV-infected women have begun to consider childbearing (VanDevanter et al., 1999). Family planning choices and experiences of heterosexual couples include unique emotional and ethical challenges and new alternatives such as sperm washing, surrogacy, and adoption depending on which gender is HIV positive (VanDevanter et al., 1999).

The relevant literature, both historic and current, has identified that couples of mixed HIV status have faced the unique and ongoing challenge of coping with the threat of transmission for one partner and the potential disease progression in the other and how these affect the couple's emotional and sexual life together (Padian et al., 1993; Rait, Ross, and Rao, 1997; Van der Straten et al., 1998; MacDonald, 1998; Remien, 1998; VanDevanter et al., 1999).

SUMMARY

The relevant literature, key authors, and researchers in this area have concurred that unique emotional challenges are indeed posed to a couple of mixed HIV status. Comparing these authors and their findings, there are clearly those issues (fear of HIV transmission, uncertainty of disease progression, disclosure issues, negotiating sexual dynamics, caregiving strains) that are shared by heterosexual and gay serodiscordant couples alike (Adam and Sears, 1994; Beckerman, Letteney, and Lorber, 2001; Foley et al., 1994; Remien, Carballo-Dieguez, and Wagner, 1995; Palmer and Bor, 2001; Powell-Cope, 1995; VanDevanter et al., 1999; Van der Straten et al., 1998). Several issues may be distinctive to gay males in serodiscordant relationships (a double stigma for sexual orientation and serostatus and a double coming out process, legal, health care, and insurance biases). For heterosexual couples of mixed HIV status, there are the unique questions of child-bearing and reproductive dilemmas. However, how HIV has impacted the desire to become parents has been articulated by gay and straight couples alike (Beckerman, Letteney, and Lorber, 2001). It is important to highlight that race, socioeconomic status, sexual orientation, gender, cultural, and spiritual aspects are central to the experiences of all individuals within their relationships and will be part of the discussion of couples of mixed HIV status throughout this book.

Chapter 3

Theoretical Framework

What informs our practice with couples of mixed HIV status? Treating any couple coping with the emotional impact of illness requires sensitivity to a variety of issues related to the past, present, and future of each unique relationship. This chapter begins with a broad overview of those theoretical orientations that have effectively informed the treatment of couples facing a wide array of relationship distresses. The second component provides a comprehensive review and analysis of theoretical approaches that can be employed effectively when treating couples coping with some commonly identified challenges precipitated by a HIV diagnosis.

Couple therapy is generally superior to individual treatment in reducing relationship distress due to a wide range of issues, including issues of psychiatric and medical illness (Alexander, Holtzworth-Munroe, and Jameson, 1994; Baucom and Hoffman, 1986; Dunn and Schweibel, 1995; Sprenkle, Blow, and Dickey, 1999). However, with the array of conjoint therapies available to a practitioner, how does one know which approaches may lend themselves better to which presenting issues and why one approach is more effective than another? Given the multifaceted uniqueness of all our clients, ourselves as practitioners, and how each of us may bring a clinical orientation to life in our practice, no one approach will always be the most effective with any one presenting complaint or issue. Yet the more we know about what couples experience with a particular set of emotional challenges precipitated by experiences with illness, the more we can begin to tailor which approaches may be best suited for such a population. Each couple coping with HIV in their relationship has a premorbid level of intrapsychic and dyadic functioning. The introduction of the HIV diagnosis into the relationship is then superimposed and can have a centrifugal effect: pushing the partners further away from one another, or a centripetal effect, pulling the partners closer together. As with any crisis, an HIV diagnosis may cause couples to simultaneously pull together in some ways and push partners apart in other ways. Before pursuing the theoretical approaches that can inform our practice with the dyadic shifts attributable to HIV, the common frameworks of couple therapy are provided as a foundation.

COMMON THEORETICAL FRAMEWORKS IN COUPLE THERAPY

A history reviewing the birth and prolific expansion of couple therapies will provide the practicing therapist with a broader context for practice with couples of mixed HIV status. These approaches emerged out of the burgeoning family systems approaches that focused primarily on parent-child relationships. In the late 1950s, behavioral modification was often the chosen framework applied to modify dysfunctional parent-child interactions and develop more adaptive parenting skills (Berkowitz and Grazing, 1972; Patterson, 1971; Stuart, 1969). During this time, family therapists began to focus traditional behavioral modification techniques to develop strategies for improving communication and behavioral interactions between distressed couples. Ellis applied the cognitive component to behavioral modification in intimate relationships (Ellis, 1977). Applying his rational emotive therapy (RET) framework to couples, Ellis included interventions that aimed to identify and modify those exaggerated or irrational beliefs and thoughts that produced negative behavioral interactions resulting in subsequent disappointment and frustration between partners (Ellis and Harper, 1961; Ellis, 1977).

Within the behavioral and cognitive marriage therapies of this era, active listening skills were greatly emphasized. This was based on the premise that couples who were able to sustain empathic communications were better equipped to establish and maintain a mutually satisfying relationship even during conflict (Jacobsen and Christensen, 1996). After extensive meta-analyses of marriage therapies, researchers concluded that active listening techniques as the centerpiece of skill development were pivotal across the myriad of marital therapies, including behavioral, systemic, communication approaches and even psychoanalytic models (Gottman, 1999; Shadish and Montgomery, 1993). Hahlweg and colleagues (1984) studied the effectiveness of active listening skills with distressed couples and concluded that although active listening showed decreases in negative interactions, a more comprehensive approach that included behavioral or emotional approaches demonstrated a decrease in negativity and an increase in positive interactions.

At the present time in its evolution, couple therapy continues to be fragmented with numerous variations stemming largely from schools of thought based in family system theories. Some of the most widely accepted of these include: behavioral marital therapy; cognitive-behavioral couple therapy; social constructionist therapy; ego-analytic therapy; experiential, feminist therapy; humanistic, Imago therapy; integrative couple therapy (ICT); medical family therapy; narrative therapy; psychodynamic therapy; solution-focused couple therapy; strategic therapy; structural therapy; transgenerational therapy; and emotionally focused couple therapy. Each of these approaches, as well as others commonly employed in couple therapy but not listed here, holds a different ideology about the nature of intimacy and the nature and source of relationship distress, and therefore, the most effective focus for clinical assessment and treatment. These numerous approaches can be conceptualized and subsumed under three fundamentally discreet approaches: behaviorally oriented, emotionally oriented, and integrated (comprised of varying components of behavioral and emotional components).

The most widely studied approaches of couple therapy have been behavioral marital therapy and its offspring, cognitive-behavioral couple therapy (Baucom et al., 1998; Gurman, Kniskern, and Pinsof, 1986). The extensive quantitative studies through the past three decades primarily measured outcomes regarding marital satisfaction. Behavioral marital therapies and cognitive behavioral marital therapies were consistently found to be effective in improving overall marital satisfaction (Dattilio, 1993, 1994; Gurman, Kniskern, and Pinsof, 1986; Gottman, 1999; Hahlweg and Markman, 1988; Hahlweg et al., 1984; Jacobsen and Addis, 1993; Jacobsen, 1991; Liberian, 1970). Subsequent research of behavioral and cognitive marital therapies indicated equally positive evaluations of these approaches (Alexander, Holtzworth-Munroe, and Jameson, 1994).

Shadish and Montgomery (1993) conducted the most wide-reaching meta-analysis of the empirical research in family and marital therapy and found that marital satisfaction was often improved for couples treated with a behavioral or cognitive-behavioral approach.

A central approach more from the behavioral orientation than insight-oriented school is structural family therapy. This is a systems approach that has historically had an emphasis on generational boundaries within systems. This approach has paid particular attention to assisting families to develop adaptive boundaries and norms, and to shoring up the executive powers of the parental subsystem (Minuchin, 1984; VonBertalanffy, 1968). Structural theory has provided theoretical and practice principles that have proved effective when working solely with the spousal subsystem in couple therapy.

A brief overview of this very rich and complex approach is provided as it can be helpful to draw on with couples of mixed HIV status. The central thesis of the structural approach developed by Minuchin (1984) is that an individual's symptoms are best understood as rooted in the context and structure of family interactions and family norms. When the structure is transformed, behaviors will shift. As behaviors shift, experiences of each other shift. Therefore, the structure of these expectations, largely unspoken, must be shifted to allow more flexibility in roles, rules, and norms that guide interactions between partners. Understanding the structure of a couple, the often invisible functional and emotional rules that dictate partners' behaviors with each other, can be particularly helpful in assessing and intervening with those couples who are not a good match for insight-oriented approaches (Epstein and Baucom, 1989).

Several key concepts are particularly relevant to couples of mixed status. The first is the concept of boundaries. It is helpful to assess first the norms concerning a couple's boundaries (the invisible demarcation between partners) and determine whether there has been a notable shift in the way a couple relates to each other and to others since the introduction of HIV in their lives (Minuchin, 1984). Minuchin (1984) posited that each system functions on a continuum of boundaries. At one end, we find a couple who is enmeshed, marked by a lack of differentiation between partners and fostering mutual overdependency between partners. On the opposite end of this continuum is the couple that has little emotional contact and lacks interdependence with each other. The therapist is assessing to what extent the boundaries that govern a couple's way of relating to each other are adaptive or maladaptive. Is this a couple that is so fused that neither partner is allowed to develop a sense of autonomy or competency, or is this a couple in which both partners experience emotional disengagement? This continuum and its flexibility is an important barometer to include when assessing the emotional attachments partners experience in their relationship and determining how an HIV diagnosis may affect these processes.

Another relevant concept basic to the structural approach is homeostasis. Each couple system maintains certain norms (such as boundaries) in ways that keep the couple emotionally and functionally stable. Homeostasis refers to those patterns and efforts that sustain the system in a state of equilibrium (Minuchin, 1984). With the diagnosis or revelation of HIV in a relationship, the couple will likely experience some level of disequilibrium. The therapist needs to assess how the couple sustained itself before the diagnosis and how the partners can adjust after the crisis and transition to a new homeostasis that includes the stress of HIV in their lives.

The assessment phase of structural therapy with couples includes attention to six areas of a couple's functioning:

1. the overall structure (including invisible norms and boundaries),
2. the flexibility of the system,
3. the capacity for sensitivity with each other,
4. the larger family life context (sources of stress, sources of support),
5. the developmental phase of a couple, and
6. use of the identified patient or symptom. (Minuchin, 1984)

Although there are numerous stages and interventions in the treatment phase of the structural approach, the three central stages of intervention have been identified by some couple therapists as joining, enactment, and unbalancing.

In joining, the therapist positions himself or herself as an approachable and accepting figure that will engage with each partner and with the system as a whole. This is particularly helpful to remember when one participant is reluctant about beginning couple therapy. Efforts need to be made to thoroughly engage the reluctant partner with the process and with the therapist. Once there is a viable therapeutic alliance and joining has been successful, a key tool in the structural approach is facilitating an in-session exhibition of how the couple interacts. This is referred to as enactment. By fostering each partner to engage with the other as they typically do around a common conflict, the therapist can learn about the unique interactional patterns he or she sees in session. Critical questions are (1) how do these patterns serve the system as a whole, and (2) are they flexible enough to change as the needs of the system changes? (Minuchin, 1984). This approach allows the therapist to assess how the couple's patterns of conflict, overfunctioning/underfunctioning, and other roles and rules serve to maintain the system as they know it, and how it can be improved to increase marital satisfaction and to foster more adaptive functioning.

To help the couple seek out and develop new interactional patterns, the old patterns have to be seen as problematic. In unbalancing, the therapist reflects the typical and problematic behavioral patterns they see and challenges those behaviors that perpetuate the dysfunction. By challenging the structural status quo of roles, rules, boundaries, and behavioral cues each partner gives to the other, the therapist unbalances the system and seeks to help the couple to limit and shift out of maladaptive functioning patterns.

These concepts and practice principles from the structural approach provide important and useful tools in assessment and intervention with couples of mixed HIV status. Overall, in a structural approach action precedes insight, as distinct from insight-oriented approaches where insight precedes action. Insight-oriented or psychodynamic models (psychoanalytic couple therapy, emotionally focused couple therapy) that are focused on the emotional experiences of the partners have been evaluated as well, and have also demonstrated positive changes in distressed relationships (Alexander, Holtzworth-Munroe, and Jameson, 1994; Baucom, Sayers, and Sheer, 1990; Greenberg and Johnson, 1988; Wile, 1995).

The postmodern school (such as brief marital therapy, solution-focused therapy, Imago therapy, social constructionist therapy, feminist therapy, and others) has not been researched systematically enough in the relevant literature to provide a substantive conclusion.

With behavioral, cognitive, and emotionally oriented approaches all proving viable, how does a therapist know which approach will be most effective with which presenting issue? Any therapeutic treatment of a couple is a multifaceted endeavor requiring the therapist to consider the impact of contributing factors to the presenting problem.

Recent meta-analyses of marriage and family therapy provide clear evidence of effectiveness for varying approaches, but found little or no substantial differences in effectiveness between the different theoretical approaches (Shadish and Montgomery, 1993; Sprenkle, Blow, and Dickey, 1999). Although research has indicated that the majority of couple therapists rely most heavily on either behavioral or insight-oriented approaches with couples in distress, no evidence exists to substantiate that either orientation is preferable (Dunn and Schweibel, 1995; Hahlweg and Markman, 1988; Shadish and Montgomery, 1993).

One of the most salient findings regarding the many different approaches used in couple therapy is not the approach itself that is at the heart of efficacy of treatment, but the confidence a couple has in their therapist, the therapist's belief that therapy is working, and the flexibility of the therapist in employing different approaches as warranted (Sprenkle, Blow, and Dickey, 1999). Indeed, the integrated approach, that is, relying on behavioral interventions where the couple has the motivation, capacity, and opportunity to work behaviorally, or applying insight-oriented interventions when the couple demonstrates the motivation and capacity for insight, provides the most successful outcome.

The combination of behavioral and emotional approaches can be tailored to meet the needs of certain couples facing a specific set of emotional and functional challenges, such as coping with physical illness (Shadish and Montgomery, 1993). In addition to crisis intervention theory and behavioral and emotionally oriented approaches, medical family therapy is a particularly relevant approach for a practitioner treating couples of mixed HIV status.

MEDICAL FAMILY THERAPY

Medical family therapy, an integration of family systems, crisis intervention, and psychoeducation, articulates the primary premise that any medical diagnosis or illness of an individual can most fully be understood as a family-oriented process (Doherty, Baird, and Becker, 1987). With the crisis of illness in an individual, the family system is often deeply affected on both a functional and emotional plane. Any threat or potential threat to the survival of one partner is a psychological threat to the other partner and their lives together. The concepts and interventions from family systems have been applied to this population quite effectively (Baider and Sarell, 1984; Campbell and Patterson, 1995; Doherty, Baird, and Becker, 1987; Gurman, Kniskern, and Pinskof, 1986).

With illness or the threat of illness comes rebalancing of the family system and the need for flexibility of roles, rules, and norms. This shake-up in norms and the emotional sequalae pertains to each challenge of illness, such as diagnosis, illness, treatment side effects, and the uncertainty and anxiety of medical illness. Medical family therapy anticipates that with the news of diagnosis the individual will experience emotional reactions, and family members will position themselves sometimes as support, sometimes as additional stressors, and sometimes as both simultaneously.

Lines of inquiry in assessment from this approach include:

1. previous nodal events around illness and how the family coped,
2. in what ways partners and family members can be drawn on to support the ill family member, and
3. the extent of need for additional support networks to aid the family.

Interventions based on medical family therapy often include:

1. advocating for patient and family to be fully educated about their health status and potential treatment alternatives,
2. facilitating open communication about the illness between family members,
3. helping the family to adjust to new functional and emotional roles, and

4. helping the patient and family to develop effective coping and adaptation to the diagnosis and illness (McDaniel, Hepworth, and Doherty, 1995).

These interventions are provided with the aim of decreasing negative behavioral interactions brought on by the anxiety of illness, improving empathic alliances between family members, and increasing the system's efficacy in coping and adaptation to chronic illness (Hahlweg et al., 1984).

In addition to medical family systems, the couple therapy approaches that can be tailored to work with couples of mixed HIV status are emotionally focused couple therapy (EFCT) and integrative couple therapy (ICT), a behaviorally based approach. EFCT and ICT have been found to be particularly effective approaches with couples facing issues commonly raised by their mixed HIV status.

EFCT AND COUPLES AFFECTED BY HIV/AIDS

When working with couples affected by HIV, therapists have often relied on the medical family systems approach, which has been effective when working with couples facing other acute or chronic illness (Winiarski, 1991; Walker, 1991). In addition to the emotional impact of illness issues, couples of mixed HIV status have to contend with an array of other unique emotional challenges that may be potentially conflictual within the relationship, such as the source of HIV and/or fear of transmission. Questions surrounding the source of the HIV transmission may result in feelings of mistrust or betrayal between partners, and the impact of preventing HIV transmission may be quite disruptive to the relationship. As the threat to one's health can sometimes be perceived as a threat to the survival of the relationship and can include such issues as betrayal and fear of abandonment, attachment theory, the insight-oriented couple theory that largely informs EFCT, is essential to a couple therapist.

Attachment theory, vis-à-vis couple therapy, focuses on the propensity for human beings to make and maintain powerful affectional bonds to significant others (Bowlby, 1988). Attachment is the bond characterized as a primary emotional interdependence between individuals and is a basic human need. A secure attachment bond is an active, affectionate, reciprocal relationship marked by emotional closeness, comfort, and security (Johnson, Makinen, and Millikin, 2001).

Attachment theory focuses on the bond between any two people in a dyad. It emphasizes the dynamics involving protection and felt security between any two individuals. The ability of the infant and growing toddler to develop a secure attachment with his or her primary caregiver, as well as to tolerate emotions provoked by separation, are the defining developmental tasks that lay the emotional blueprint for all future relationships. According to Bowlby (1969, 1988), adaptive attachment (attachments marked by security and trust) is the essential building block of adaptive personality development and the capacity for adaptive adult relationships.

Bowlby (1969) described four different types of attachment dynamics: secure, avoidant, ambivalent, and disorganized. These classifications have helped to explain both caregiver-infant attachment dynamics as well as adult attachment dynamics. The affectional resonance of primary relationships (referred to as the internalized object) is the primary arbiter of dynamic patterns repeated in adult intimate relationships, and those who do not have adaptive experiences in primary attachments are more vulnerable to the emotional extremes in adult relationships, for example, chronically ambivalent, isolated, or enmeshed (Bowlby, 1988). Although attachment theory has been used historically to better understand how this bond is created between mother and child, recent research has applied it to better understand the attachment issues that manifest in adult relationships (Feeney, 1999). Indeed, we often see that partners are replicating the primary attachment dynamics of their formative years with their partners (Johnson and Greenberg, 1995). Attachment classifications such as secure, ambivalent, avoidant, and disorganized have been used to further understand and intervene with the latent dynamics of maladaptive transactional patterns and chronic conflicts of couples in relationship distress (Johnson and Greenberg, 1995; Johnson, 1988). The adult attachment style deeply affects the couple's functioning and is particularly relevant in the light of illness or the potential for illness in one partner. With such a threat facing the couple, attachment issues around insecurity, betrayal, and abandonment may manifest as the security of the bond is challenged (Johnson, Makinen, and Millikin, 2001).

This theoretical framework asserts that profound emotions of fear, anger, and sadness will result if an attachment figure is experienced as inaccessible or unresponsive (Johnson, 1988). Further, this framework helps us to understand the common dynamic with couples in which the more one partner withdraws (threatening the attachment) the more the other partner clings to regain the security of the attachment bond. Some relationships progress toward chronic disengagement as each partner emotionally withdraws in response to the perceived withdrawal of their partner.

Attachment theory is a particularly useful framework to understand couples in conflict because often the underlying emotions contributing to the conflict involve the specter of a break in the attachment, a perceived betrayal or abandonment (Johnson and Greenberg, 1995). As Bowlby (1969) has posited, individual partners create and replicate the relationship based on their formative attachment experiences and beliefs about attachment. Those who have experienced insecure attachments may anticipate the same type of experience, and position themselves in ways that re-create and repeat insecure attachments. In adult romantic attachments, each partner is an attachment figure, and in bonding, each partner is provided with varying levels of security.

Assessing the nature of each unique attachment has to include sensitivity to the unique experiences of sexual orientation, culture, religion, and the role of gender. As so many couples of mixed HIV status are gay male couples, it is critical to note that "whatever their sexual orientation, individuals have strong needs to attach to others and to form intimate relationships" (Mohr, 1999, p. 83). For gay male couples, the therapist has to pay different attention to the ways in which men have been socialized to form attachments.

Greenan and Tunnell (2003) make excellent contributions to our understanding of which factors are the same and which are different when focusing on attachments in gay male couples. Key among these contributions is the conceptualization of attachment between adult partners, the continuum between the evaluation of autonomy as a preferred state (Bowen's 1978 cornerstone concept of healthy differentiation), and dependency as a nonpathologized sign of health (Bowlby's 1988 position that attachment is not a stage to be outgrown, but a normative state in all individuals). As many family theories have evolved, it has become evident that the healthy state for a family or couple is one in which attachments provide a balance of both dependency and autonomy differentially. This is particularly relevant to gay male couples of mixed HIV status, as often conflict exists about the nature and viability of the attachment in the face of medical crisis. In addition, issues of independence versus dependence on the part of the HIV-positive partner may be experienced differently in same-sex attachments than in heterosexual partnerships.

Greenan and Tunnell (2003) explore and explain that issues of emotional intimacy may play out with different obstacles in gay male relationships than in heterosexual relationships. Important factors to consider are gender roles (or lack thereof), difficulty expressing feelings of vulnerability and difficulty tolerating an intimate nurturing attachment from another man due to their own internalized homophobia.

Without the rigid societal expectations of gender-specific roles, gay male couples (and lesbian couples) must develop their own authentic set of norms about functional and emotional roles and demands in the relationship. As men have been socialized to value independence and autonomy, it may be generally more difficult to express vulnerability or dependency. Men have not been socialized to express their dependency needs or vulnerable feelings, and certainly not with other men. Another important component to consider is that most gay men have grown up "keeping their emotional lives private from others" (Greenan and Tunnell, 2003, p. 27). This must be considered in assessing the complexities of two men in an intimate relationship who may have trained themselves not to attach in full and open ways. Because we live in a heterosexist society and a culture that prizes heterosexuality and marginalizes (at best) and demonizes (at worst) homosexuality, it is not uncommon that some gay men may experience varying levels of shame, guilt, or discomfort with their own needs (St. Lawrence et al., 1990). This deeply affects their ability to create and enjoy a successful, satisfying gay male attachment.

Gay men, like heterosexual men, have been acculturated to be more rational than emotional, independence being a sign of strength and dependence being a sign of weakness. How then do they cope with loss, illness, and injury and how are their partners expected to cope and respond? In addition, many gay men have experienced multiple losses due to their sexual orientation and/or HIV/AIDS (Neugenberger et al., 1992). Theorists purport that men tend to withhold their emotional experiences of hurt and loss and women tend to express these vulnerable emotions more easily (Gilligan, 1982).

The couple, whether gay or heterosexual will experience myriad emotional reactions to the HIV diagnosis that may exacerbate preexisting dyadic conflicts and underlying attachment issues (VanDevanter et al., 1999). Johnson, Makinen, and Milliken (2001) introduces the construct of attachment injury. The negative attachment-related events (abandonment and betrayal) often cause pervasive and lingering damage. Attachment injury is conceptualized as a wound that occurs when one partner fails to emotionally respond to the other, and the event then continues to be used as an obstacle to intimacy in the clinical process.

This is a dynamic wherein injuries reemerge in therapy and are compounded when the partner is not able to repair the break in the couple's empathic connection. The usefulness of attachment theory is in the premise that we relate to our partners in adult intimate relationships based largely on perceptions of self and other formed by early attachments. The premise proffers that with motivation, capacity, and opportunity one can therefore learn how to modify attachment behaviors.

If one conceptualizes the diagnosis of HIV as an injury to the security of the emotional bond between partners, EFCT is quite responsive to unspoken and underlying interpersonal conflicts regarding serodiscordance in relationships. EFCT focuses on reestablishing the positive primary attachment in order to regain positive empathic alliances between partners (Johnson and Greenberg, 1995). EFCT has been effective with couples presenting with issues of abuse, conflict, and the crisis of chronic physical illness (Johnson and Williams-Keeler, 1998). The focus of EFCT is on how to help couples regain, maintain, or achieve a secure emotional bond. One component of the premise of EFCT is that a secure emotional bond helps people to cope better with the crisis of physical illness. EFCT creates and/or facilitates sustained adaptive changes because it integrates intrapsychic and interpersonal factors and redefines the attachment bonds between

partners at a time they need each other the most. Of utmost importance is the ability to sustain emotional engagement throughout illness (Johnson and Williams-Keeler, 1998).

This approach has demonstrated significant clinical effectiveness
in facilitating more positive aspects of intimate relationships (Dunn
and Schweibel, 1995; Johnson et al., 1999). With family-of-origin
work, partners will benefit from increased emotional clarity regarding the impact that early attachments may have on their adult intimate
relationships when faced with HIV/AIDS.

Assessment

The therapist who is informed by EFCT will not focus on the content, but on the affectional significance of their clients' attachment to
each other. The two goals of EFCT are to "access and reprocess the
emotional experiences of partners," and to "restructure interaction
patterns" (Johnson and Greenberg, 1995, p. 127). As the therapist facilitates articulation of underlying emotions about the attachment,
fear of abandonment, and ambivalence about the existential conflict
of simultaneously needing dependence and independence in the relationship, the partners are assisted to empathize with unspoken primary emotions.

Johnson and Greenberg (1995) explain that as partners experience
their primary emotions and voice them in session, they encounter new
aspects of themselves and each other, and are then more able to increasingly develop functional interaction patterns that are aimed at
satisfying their attachment needs. The primary goal is to repair the intimate emotional bond, enabling the partners to become engaged
emotionally so that they are more able to respond to each other's underlying attachment needs (Johnson, 1999).

This approach includes nine steps or interventions that are commonly employed:

1. delineating conflict issues in the core struggle (where the therapist assesses the conflicting issues presented);
2. identifying negative interaction cycles (how each partner contributes to the transactional patterns that have become negative);

3. accessing the unacknowledged feelings and underlying inter-actional positions, (assisting the partners to identify and own feelings that contribute to the perpetuation of the transactional patterns);
4. reframing the problem in terms of underlying feelings/attach-ment needs (translating the conflictual behavioral and commu-nication patterns to shed light on emotional needs);
5. identifying disowned needs and aspects of self and integrating these into relationship interactions;
6. promoting acceptance of the partner's experiences and new in-teraction patterns;
7. facilitating experience of needs/wants and creating emotional engagement (helping partners to articulate their emotional needs and helping them to build an empathic connection;
8. establishing the emergence of new solutions; and
9. consolidating new emotional and therefore behavioral positions in relation to each other (Johnson and Greenberg, 1995).

Through the use of dyadic interpretation and facilitation, along with insight-oriented exploration and interpretations, partners can be assisted in empathizing with each other's attachment conflicts and developing a different appreciation for each other's struggles. This in turn helps couples develop more adaptive behavioral interactions re-garding coping with HIV in their relationship (Beckerman and Auer-bach, 2002).

A combination of insight-oriented approaches with some cogni-tive behavioral interventions has proven particularly effective for couples living with the emotional impact of physical illness (Camp-bell and Patterson, 1995). This brings us to integrative couple therapy (ICT) and its role in treatment of couples of mixed HIV status.

INTEGRATIVE COUPLE THERAPY
WITH COUPLES AFFECTED BY HIV/AIDS

When couples of mixed HIV status seek therapy, typically there are conflicts that appear unrelated, as well as those directly related to the HIV diagnosis. Commonly, those behaviors or personality differences that were manageable before the HIV diagnosis become more problematic after diagnosis. Issues such as shifts in emotional intimacy or feelings of mistrust may or may not have been integral to the fabric of a couple before HIV, but commonly appear with full force in response to HIV. Issues such as fear of HIV transmission, coping with uncertainty of illness, disclosure of HIV status outside of the relationship, and obstacles to having children are now added to preexisting conflicts. To provide only insight or only behaviorally oriented interventions is to confine the therapeutic process unnecessarily. As helpful as emotionally focused couple therapy can be, there are some issues and some couples who will respond more easily and more successfully to behaviorally oriented interventions, as long as both partners are thoroughly engaged emotionally.

Integrative couple therapy (ICT) is an approach that stemmed primarily from traditional behavioral marital therapy, but combines the emotionally oriented component of empathy and acceptance that is central to emotionally focused couple therapy. The premise of traditional behavioral couple therapy has been that by shifting aversive behaviors of each partner to a more desired set of behaviors, couples will experience improved marital satisfaction. With the development of active listening skills and problem-solving skills, couples can be helped to identify and articulate those behaviors in each partner that are experienced as conflictual and even, at times, intolerable. However, for those couples that are experiencing acute conflict (marked by anger and frustration), the motivation necessary for traditional behavioral marital therapy has not always been present. Intervening solely on a behavioral plane excludes the very real scenario that commonly occurs between distressed couples; emotions of anger or despair that are experienced so intensely that the couple is rendered incapable of shifting targeted behaviors.

When behavioral interventions become obstructed by underlying emotions, ICT recommends that attention be paid to the emotional conflicts that are part of undesired behaviors and the partners' inability to accept each other. ICT has a dual focus which aims to (1) shift aversive behaviors, and (2) facilitate emotional acceptance of vexing behaviors. Interventions are focused toward promoting intimacy and tolerance of each other's needs and behavioral styles. The change then takes place in both partners; the partner who shifts his or her behavior, and the partner who shifts his or her reaction to the unwanted behaviors. To help the couple reach these goals ICT facilitates better communication and problem-solving skills so that partners can artic-ulate what the undesired behaviors are, as well as their emotional re-action to them. This integrated approach attempts to strengthen rela-tionship skills to enable behavior changes and acceptance, but also to foster intimacy (Jacobsen, 1991). The intimacy is a byproduct of helping partners to better understand and empathize with the emo-tional experiences of each other's undesirable or hurtful behaviors. With this emotional intimacy, the improved dynamic will be marked by increased motivation for both partners to shift behaviors and both to be more accepting. An important premise of ICT is quite naturalis-tic and common sense: if the dynamic can result in increased marital satisfaction for both, they will be more likely to repeat it. As behav-iors shift toward more positive interactions for both, emotional satis-faction increases. This emphasis on behavioral changes and accep-tance of behaviors dovetails with the essence of empathic joining that is at the heart of EFCT.

Another intervention in ICT is the emotional detachment from the conflict. With communication skills honed, couples are assisted to disengage from typical accusatory stances and move toward sharing the conflict together. By working with both partners to take responsi-bility and avoid blame, to understand the circular nature of dynamics in couples and to release their blaming positioning, the couples can experience the problem as something to be tackled together. Baucom and Epstein (1990) explain, "Ideally, the couple begins to see the problem as something they both share, not something the other is re-sponsible for" (p. 108). The emphasis is much like EFCT, repairing the elemental bond between the partners that underlies the disruptive behaviors. Whether focusing on behavior changes, emotional accep-tance, or unified detachment from the problem, ICT can be applied differentially to a variety of presenting issues as diverse as shifts in emotional and sexual intimacy, such as those often present in couples of mixed HIV status (Jacobsen and Christensen, 1996b).

When practicing from an integrative approach, the unique needs of the couple and intuitions of the practitioner will define the emphasis placed on behavior change interventions versus emotional accep-tance interventions, but to have both at one's disposal has proven to be more effective than either approach alone (Jacobsen and Christensen, 1996b).

SUMMARY

Essential clinical interventions borrowed from crisis intervention theory, medical family therapy, and emotionally and behaviorally oriented approaches can be applied effectively to the issues commonly confronting couples of mixed HIV status. The unique needs, motivations, and capacities of each couple will be the ultimate arbiter of which theoretical framework might be best suited for each couple. With this in mind, the practitioner will need to understand the couple's preexisting emotional and behavioral patterns and how they may be exacerbated by the HIV diagnosis. Although there may be effective application of a multitude of other couple therapies, medical family therapy EFCT and ICT can be used effectively in assessment and treatment of couples coping with HIV in their relationship.

Chapter 4

Methodology

This chapter provides an overview of the quantitative design of the empirical research, as well as an overview of the qualitative data based on case material from clinical practice. The cases do not represent respondents from the empirical study—they are cases from clinical practice that have been duly disguised. Both methods are introduced and placed in the context of the study area: identifying the common emotional challenges of couples of mixed HIV status.

EMPIRICAL STUDY

Research Strategy

The goal of this study was to identify and clarify the unique emotional challenges confronting couples of mixed HIV status in the era of combination therapies. The study was exploratory in order to gather a range of information about a subject not previously researched. With the use of open-ended questions, the author could better identify trends as well as frequencies of emotional issues facing couples of mixed HIV status.

Characteristics of Participating Partners

This sample, based on eighty-eight individuals in forty-four serodiscordant couples, represented demographic diversity including (1) HIV-positive and HIV-negative individuals in serodiscordant relationships, (2) inclusion of women, (3) heterosexual and homosexual individuals, and d) diversity in ethnicity.

HIV-Positive and HIV-Negative Sample Representation

The sample consists of forty-four HIV-positive individuals and their respective HIV-negative partners. The sample and the break-down by gender, sexual orientation, ethnicity, and serostatus is provided in the following list:

Gender
Female   20
Male   68

Sexual Orientation
Straight   40
Gay   48

Ethnicity
White   37
Hispanic   28
Black   21

HIV Status
HIV+   44
HIV-   44

The average length of the relationships that comprise this discussion are also important. The majority (n = 28 couples) of the couples have been together for an average of seven years. Sixteen couples have been together less than seven years. This allows for a new view into long-term established relationships that HIV has intruded upon.

There is an equal distribution between those couples who have experienced their first HIV-related illness (n = 26), and those couples who have not experienced a HIV-related illness (n = 18), thus providing the opportunity to understand how a couple experiences the emergence of illness. These diverse sample characteristics combine to provide a unique and compelling view of the common psychosocial tasks and coping patterns among serodiscordant couples.

Recruitment of Participants

The criteria for participation was to be currently involved in a primary emotional relationship in which one partner has tested HIV positive and the other has tested negative. Preliminary discussions were held with HIV/AIDS social workers and social work supervisors who provided psychotherapy and case management to clients living with HIV/AIDS who were known to be currently in a primary relationship with a partner who was seronegative.

The sample was collected from seventeen metropolitan and suburban sites in the United States, comprised of nine outpatient hospitals and eleven community-based AIDS support organizations. Each site reviewed its caseload and identified individuals in serodiscordant couples who met the criteria for the study. One hundred and fifty questionnaires were distributed in all. The time frame was one year, from mid-2001 to mid-2002.

Instrument

A pilot instrument was built on themes identified in existing literature, e.g., fear of HIV transmission, uncertainty, anxiety and depression, stigma, and disclosure within serodiscordant couples (Shelby, 1992; Powell-Cope, 1995; Remien, 1998; Williams-Saporito, 1998), as well as several interviews with key witnesses who provide HIV/AIDS counseling and HIV/AIDS couple counseling to serodiscordant couples. The pilot responses confirmed the presence of these issues and also indicated issues related to reproduction (primarily among heterosexual couples), caregiving, emotional intimacy, and emotional distancing.

A Likert scale consisting of twenty-five items and coded on a four-point range from "strongly agree" to "strongly disagree" was developed for the study. The scale sought to measure the psychosocial issues common to individuals in serodiscordant relationships. Some of the key questions asked were to what degree fear of HIV transmission was of primary concern, to what degree HIV-related uncertainty impacted their relationship, to what degree HIV made them emotionally closer or more distant, to what degree HIV impacted their decisions about having children, to what degree HIV caused their family/friends to respond with stigma, to what degree HIV was at the center of their conflicts, etc.

The questionnaire also included five open-ended questions to avoid fixed responses and allow for more range and exploration. Each respondent was asked (1) to identify key HIV-related emotional issues in his or her relationship, (2) how HIV has brought the couple emotionally closer, (3) how HIV has made the couple more emotionally distant, (4) how would their lives be different if one of them did not have HIV, and (5) how HIV has affected their decisions regarding reproduction.

These are the scale and open-ended items that relate to the themes identified in the literature regarding serodiscordant relationships, key witnesses, and the pilot instrument. The distribution and collection of the data was done by this author.

Data Analysis

Based on responses from all 88 subjects, significant trends and patterns emerged. The Likert responses were analyzed with a univariate method in order to identify the frequencies; i.e., which emotional issues were most commonly experienced by serodiscordant couples. The responses to the five open-ended questions were analyzed with content analysis to identify trends.

QUALITATIVE RESEARCH

Qualitative data can be based on observation and interviews over a sustained period of time in order to better describe and analyze relationships and dynamics (Merriam, 2002). Observation in clinical experience yields a different form of data that can complement the empirical portion of research. It is important to include qualitative data as this focuses on naturally occurring events, that is, capturing real-life behaviors and feelings (Merriam, 2002). With the emphasis on people's lived experiences, qualitative data offer wider breadth and depth in our attempt to understand and appreciate the complex dynamics of how people interact verbally and nonverbally. This form of analysis lends itself quite well in identifying how emotional challenges might truly impact and manifest in couples of mixed HIV status.

Conceptual and clinical insights are gleaned from ongoing case material (duly disguised) from clinical practice. Multiple cases offer the researcher an even deeper understanding of the processes and dynamics between partners. Several couples will be introduced and followed through Chapters 6 to 11 to further illustrate the range of emotional issues and dynamics that have been witnessed and intervened with in clinical practice. These couples were not part of the sample of the empirical study, but were seen in clinical practice. There are instances in which clinical practice with couples of mixed HIV status yielded insights and patterns that concur with the findings of the empirical study, and there are other instances in which conflict exists between the two forms of data. The qualitative data are included to provide the broadest range as well as the most accurate representation of the types of emotional issues and challenges that may commonly arise.

Limitations and Generalizability

Several potential limitations of this study may affect the generalizabilty of the findings. The primary limitation is that only those couples who were particularly motivated to take the time to respond did so. The small number of the sample limits its generalizability. Another limitation is that the sample represents those individuals who are already connected to the social service network by receiving HIV/AIDS counseling. Those individuals without access to medical or mental health services may present with differing experiences altogether. The limitation inherent in the qualitative data analysis is the inevitable bias that is part of the interpretation of the researcher. The researcher may interpret and generalize qualitative data based on his or her own personal and professional value base. The potential lack of generalizability of this study calls for future research of a larger sample of couples of mixed HIV status, and more fully representative of diverse geographical regions. The next chapter introduces the key and secondary findings.

Chapter 5

Introduction to the Findings

EMPIRICAL FINDINGS

A range of emotional challenges and conflicts are commonly experienced by couples of mixed HIV status. Based on the research study outlined in the previous chapter, six primary emotional issues were identified. This chapter introduces these six emotional issues:

1. fear of HIV transmission,
2. shifts in emotional intimacy,
3. coping with uncertainty,
4. disclosure issues,
5. issues of mistrust and betrayal, and
6. HIV and family planning.

A brief overview of critical findings is provided in Table 5.1, and the empirical and anecdotal responses, as well as case summaries, are presented in detail throughout the remainder of the book.

Impact of Fear of HIV Transmission

Fear of HIV transmission was the primary issue respondents strongly agreed with as the emotional issue most affecting their relationships. Eighty-three percent (n = 73) reported strong concern about HIV transmission within their relationship. Within and across categories of serostatus, sexual orientation, and gender all respondents considered fear of HIV transmission as the primary concern. Variations among gender, ethnicity, sexual orientation, and serostatus will be identified and discussed. Respondents identified and described a range of ways that their fear of HIV transmission has affected their lives together. Several couples from different backgrounds

TABLE 5.1. Overview of key findings.

	Strongly agree	Agree	Disagree	Strongly disagree
Fear of HIV transmission	83% (n = 73)	17% (n = 15)		
Emotional intimacy changes	70% (n = 62)	21% (n = 18)	9% (n = 8)	
Uncertainty	69% (n = 61)	22% (n = 19)	9% (n = 8)	
Disclosure	33% (n = 29)	35% (n = 31)	26% (n = 23)	6% (n = 5)
Mistrust/betrayal	22% (n = 19)	27% (n = 24)	26% (n = 23)	25% (n = 22)
Family planning	14% (n = 12)	15% (n = 13)	44% (n = 39)	27% (n = 24)

will be presented to illustrate how this issue may affect the couple's life together. These issues and their implications for practice are fully explored and analyzed in the following chapter.

Emotional Intimacy

Seventy percent (n = 62) reported that they strongly agreed that significant shifts occurred in their emotional intimacy due to the impact of HIV on their relationship. A surprising trend was the significant amount of anecdotal reports that clarified that the larger shift was the increased emotional intimacy as a result of one partner testing HIV positive. At the same time, respondents also identified a trend that emotional distancing occurred more intensely since the HIV diagnosis. The trends and nuances of shifts in emotional intimacy among heterosexual and homosexual couples, men and women, and different ethnic backgrounds in HIV-discordant relationships will be discussed fully in Chapter 7.

Impact of Uncertainty

Sixty-nine percent (n = 61) identified uncertainty as a primary emotional challenge. This was the consistent pattern across sexual orientation and gender. Respondents described an anxious uncertainty that has been referred to in AIDS literatures as the sword of Damocles. The couple lives with a sense that their situation is forever precarious, that they are always waiting for their lives to be changed by an HIV/AIDS-related infection at any time. There is a constant experience of anticipating the worst case scenario, and yet hoping that an infection does not emerge. There is also the uncertainty that medications that have kept viral loads low may no longer be effective or may cause intolerable side effects. These are some of the uncertainties that have been identified. Variations among gender, ethnicity, sexual orientation, and serostatus, case illustrations, and implications for couple therapy are discussed in Chapter 8.

Disclosure

Thirty-three percent (n = 29) strongly agreed that issues surrounding to whom they disclose the positive HIV status, along with when and how, created significant conflict within the relationship. This was more prevalent among heterosexuals than homosexuals, more prevalent among males than females, and more prevalent among African Americans and Hispanics than white respondents.

The length of time the couple has been together and when they learned the HIV diagnosis of one partner has many implications. When a partner has had time to integrate his or her reaction to being HIV positive individually, prior to establishing a relationship, it appears to be significantly less conflictual for the overall relationship than when both learn of the HIV diagnosis at the same time. Less divisive implications surround the HIV-positive partner's source of HIV transmission—when a partner is diagnosed in an established, monogamous relationship, there are immediate repercussions as this may be seen as evidence of sexual activity outside of the relationship. The complexities of this issue, how it manifested in couples therapy, and recommendations on how to work with it are offered in detail in Chapter 9.

Issues of Mistrust and Betrayal

Twenty-two percent (n = 19) of the respondents reported that their relationship was affected occasionally by issues of mistrust and betrayal around the source of HIV. Persistent concerns existed around either nonmonogamous relationships or bisexual or gay activities among heterosexual couples. Examples of how these feelings and suspicions affected various relationships are discussed in full detail in Chapter 10.

Family Planning

Fourteen percent (n = 12) of individuals reported that they and their partners have been deeply affected by HIV in their relationship as it impinges on their desire to have children. For some respondents, they and their partners share in a desire to have children and are wary about passing HIV on to their partner or baby. Other respondents describe ongoing conflict in their relationship because partners feel differently about HIV and family planning. The findings, narrative illustrations, and couple therapy implications are provided and reviewed in depth in Chapter 11.

QUALITATIVE DATA

To more fully understand the breadth and depth of emotional experiences that diverse couples of mixed HIV status are faced with, the responses to open-ended questions will be included throughout the text. Where notable trends emerged from the narrative responses, they will be highlighted. In some instances, the responses amplify the statistical findings; in other cases they shed a different light on what emerged statistically. In both cases, they bring a more human face to these emotional experiences.

Case presentations will be included to further elucidate how the same issue may manifest differently depending on characterological and cultural factors. The cases do not represent respondents from within the empirical study, but are composite cases from clinical practice duly disguised. Issues of difference and commonality among couples in therapy, as well as issues of transference and countertransference will be included. A conceptual framework based largely on practice principles from emotionally focused couple therapy and integrative couple therapy are applied with each case study.

Chapter 6

Fear of HIV Transmission

I long to be with him again, even just to be held, but he's afraid
to get the virus.

OVERVIEW

Once a partner has tested HIV positive, life will never resume as it
was. This has been referred to as *life after diagnosis* or *life A.D.*
Although this term was coined in the earlier stages of the HIV/AIDS
epidemic, it is not thoroughly outdated or inaccurate. Each individual
and each couple are faced with emotional challenges related to accepting and adapting to the reality and the fantasies around HIV being present in their lives.

One particular set of challenges revolves around the transmission
of HIV. The spoken and, more often, unspoken fears and anxieties between partners about becoming infected by HIV and infecting one's
loved one with HIV were consistently identified as primary sources
of concern. In empirical findings, narrative responses, and case material, couples of mixed HIV status overwhelmingly identified fear of
HIV transmission as a primary concern in their relationship.

Anxieties and fears surrounding transmission manifested themselves in myriad ways, and of course, in both overt and hidden dynamics particular to each couple. Nevertheless, some level of disruption was uniformly experienced as this fear presented itself in a
couple's emotional and sexual relationship. The most direct implica-
tion of these fears emerged in a couple's sexual relationship. With the
fear of transmission, couples often experienced the interruption of
their previous sexual life and norms. Each partner within each couple

had unique challenges and emotional responses that can be understood across a continuum. Some experienced denial, marked by a couple's complete avoidance of the issue. On the other extreme, some couples experienced endless discussions about safer sex practices that resulted in power struggles and conflict, i.e., who is in power of preventing HIV transmission and how is this power shared. With these two dynamics as end points on the continuum, partners' emotional struggles with each other were found at either end, anywhere in the middle, and fluctuating.

QUANTITATIVE FINDINGS

When asked whether fear of HIV transmission was a primary concern in their relationship, 83 percent (n = 73) of respondents strongly agreed. Seventeen percent (n = 15) agreed. No respondents disagreed. The many ways in which this fear affected relationships are expanded on by the narrative responses and the cases later in this chapter. The slight variations across sexual orientation, gender, ethnicity, and serostatus are provided in Table 6.1.

Table 6.1 illustrates the slight differential between those couples who identify themselves as heterosexual and homosexual. Heterosexual couples appear to have experienced more emotional difficulty with fear of HIV transmission than their homosexual counterparts. Thirty out of forty heterosexuals strongly agreed that fear of HIV transmission within their relationship was of primary concern, whereas thirty-five out of forty-eight homosexuals strongly agreed that fear of HIV transmission was of primary concern in their relationships. This variation indicates that the fear of HIV transmission

TABLE 6.1. Sexual orientation: Fear of HIV transmission is of primary concern.

	Strongly agree	Agree	Disagree	Strongly disagree	Total
Heterosexual	38 (95%)	2 (5%)	0	0	40
Homosexual	35 (73%)	13 (27%)	0	0	48

may be somewhat more likely to strongly affect a heterosexual relationship than a homosexual relationship.

This may be explained by several sociopolitical hypotheses. The gay community has been involved more effectively with safer sex training, prevention, and education. In fact, many venues of HIV/AIDS prevention are central to the culture of the gay community on both a formal and informal level (Green, 1995). Hence, their acceptance and understanding of safer sex practices, and therefore their level of fear of HIV transmission is somewhat lower.

Another supposition that has been supported by relevant literature explains that men (whether gay or straight) often feel more empowered (though certainly not always) in their sexual relationships than do their female counterparts (Beckerman, Letteney, and Lorber, 2001; Bromberg et al., 1991; Gillman and Newman, 1996; Goldstein, 1997). Women in serodiscordant heterosexual relationships are at higher risk for acquiring HIV than their male counterparts in heterosexual relationships, and have consistently struggled to require or even request that their male partners abide by safer sex precautions (Cates and Stone, 1992; Denenberg, 1990; Klitzman, 1997). This is further demonstrated in the findings regarding gender and fear of HIV transmission in Table 6.2.

One would have anticipated a more significant variation between males and females in heterosexual relationships, yet this finding does support that more females strongly agree that fear of HIV transmission is a primary concern in their relationship. Women tend to experience more anxiety about fear of HIV transmission regardless of who is infected in their relationship. This can also be explained by women feeling more at risk of transmission than male partners, as well as cultural influences that may contribute to many women feeling passive

TABLE 6.2. Gender in heterosexual relationships: Fear of HIV transmission is of primary concern.

	Strongly agree	Agree	Disagree	Strongly disagree	Total
Female	20 (100%)	0	0	0	20
Male	16 (80%)	4 (20%)	0	0	20
Total	36	4	0	0	40

about negotiating their HIV concerns (Beckerman, 2000; Mayer and Wells, 1997; Moore et al., 1995). A further look at how this issue affected males and females within heterosexual relationships with the variation of their respective serostatus is provided in Table 6.3.

Interestingly, women with HIV agreed more strongly that fear of HIV transmission affected their relationship than their male counterparts who were HIV positive. This is the converse for males whose reported fear of HIV transmission was consistently higher when they were the HIV-negative partner than when they were the HIV-positive partner. This is consistent with anecdotal and empirical literature on serodiscordance in heterosexual relationships, which indicates that when the female is HIV positive, she is more preoccupied with protecting her male partner than the reverse (Williams-Saporito, 1998). This phenomenon can be explained by the cultural norms of gender roles that often proscribe women as caregivers, with a primary responsibility for the well-being of their partners and families.

Although there was strong agreement overall that fear of HIV transmission is an issue that affected couples' lives together, there was a slight variation from one ethnicity to another.

Table 6.4 is based on the individual's ethnic identity and therefore does not illuminate those couples who identified as interracial. The responses from the entire sample demonstrate that within each ethnicity, fear of HIV transmission is a primary area of concern. African-

TABLE 6.3. HIV-positive partners in heterosexual relationships: Fear of HIV transmission is of primary concern.

	Strongly agree	Agree	Disagree	Strongly disagree	Total
HIV-positive women	8 (80%)	0	2 (20%)	0	10
HIV-positive men	2 (20%)	2 (20%)	4 (40%)	2 (20%)	10
HIV-negative women	2 (20%)	6 (60%)	2 (20%)	0	10
HIV-negative men	8 (80%)	2 (20%)	0	0	10
Total	20	10	8	2	40

American respondents appeared to have been somewhat more troubled than Hispanic and white respondents appeared to be. Overall, these were small variations that do not indicate any particular trend or pattern regarding ethnicity and fear of HIV transmission.

A small variation emerged within the sample between HIV-positive and HIV-negative partners. Fear of HIV transmission was strongly identified more frequently by HIV-negative partners (n = 41) than by HIV-positive partners (n = 32) as seen in Table 6.5.

Secondary Quantitative Findings

Several other noteworthy variables include the length of the relationship and the presence of HIV-related illness. There was a correlative connection between length of relationship and fear of HIV trans-

TABLE 6.4. Ethnicity: Fear of HIV transmission is of primary concern.

	Strongly agree	Agree	Disagree	Strongly disagree	Total
African American	22 (96%)	1 (4%)	0	0	23
Hispanic	22 (79%)	6 (21%)	0	0	28
White	29 (78%)	8 (22%)	0	0	37
Total	73	15	0	0	88

TABLE 6.5. Serostatus: Fear of HIV transmission is of primary concern.

	Strongly agree	Agree	Disagree	Strongly disagree	Total
HIV positive	32 (73%)	12 (27%)	0	0	44
HIV negative	41 (93%)	3 (7%)	0	0	44
Total	73	15	0	0	88

mission within the relationship. The longer the relationship, the less fear of HIV transmission affected the relationship. Fifty-six individuals reported that they had been in this present relationship for more than five years. Thirty-two individuals reported that their relationship has been less than five years.

This trend is confirmed by analysis of qualitative responses, in which one sees that the longer a couple has been together, the better equipped they may be to absorb and cope with the emotional impact of HIV diagnosis (Table 6.6). Coping mechanisms appear to be more firmly in place the longer the relationship has been maintained, but this is not to imply that their coping mechanisms are always adaptive. For some, this is one more injury to the relationship that has been maintained by denial, hence the low anxiety about fear of transmission.

For some, the HIV diagnosis comes after a series of revelations of substance abuse, sexual activity outside the relationship, and for heterosexual couples, bisexual or homosexual activity outside of the relationship. For others the HIV diagnosis comes all at once, unfolding numerous secrets such as substance abuse, sexual activity outside of the relationship, and bisexual or homosexual behaviors that have been engaged in unbeknownst to the heterosexual partner. An interesting variable to understand as practitioners is whether a difference exists in the emotional challenges being serodiscordant poses for those couples that knew of their mixed HIV status as they entered into a relationship versus those couples who had to adjust to this shift after the relationship had been formed (Table 6.7). As one might imagine, those couples who started their courtship aware of their mixed HIV

TABLE 6.6. Length of relationship: Fear of HIV transmission is of primary concern.

	Strongly agree	Agree	Disagree	Strongly disagree	Total
Less than 5 years	32 (100%)	0	0	0	32
More than 5 years	41 (73%)	15 (27%)	0	0	56
Total	73	15	0	0	88

TABLE 6.7. When couple learned of HIV diagnosis: Fear of HIV transmission is of primary concern.

	Strongly agree	Agree	Disagree	Strongly disagree	Total
Diagnosed before relationship	16 (67%)	8 (33%)	0	0	24
Diagnosed in relationship	57 (89%)	7 (11%)	0	0	64
Total	73	15	0	0	88

status fared somewhat better than those who had to incorporate and adjust individually and as a couple to an array of emotional reactions associated with HIV diagnosis.

Finally, for those couples who had experienced HIV-related illnesses versus those who had not, there are different levels of concern regarding fear of transmission. Of fifty-two respondents who reported their relationship had experienced HIV-related illness, thirty-seven respondents strongly agreed that fear of HIV transmission has affected their relationship. For those serodiscordant couples who have not experienced HIV-related illness, 100 percent (n = 36) strongly agreed that fear of HIV transmission affected their relationship (Table 6.8).

Overall, HIV-positive partners in both heterosexual and homosexual relationships appear to feel quite strongly that fear of HIV transmission greatly affected their relationships. The range of ways in which couples are impacted by this fear and anxiety are illustrated in the respondents' narrative responses to open-ended questions.

QUALITATIVE FINDINGS

Responses to Open-Ended Questions

The narrative responses expanded the ways in which this anxiety affects couples' day-to-day functional and emotional lives together in the present and in the anticipated future. The most common narrative

TABLE 6.8. HIV-related illness: Fear of HIV transmission is of primary concern.

	Strongly agree	Agree	Disagree	Strongly disagree	Total
Have had HIV illness	37 (71%)	15 (29%)	0	0	52
Have not had HIV illness	36 (100%)	0	0	0	36
Total	73	15	0	0	88

response reinforced the centrality of this issue for couples of mixed HIV status from both viewpoints.

> "Ever since I tested positive, I just can't get past that I could infect her. I worry about it all the time, and feel terrible about it. She thinks I've lost interest, but I don't want her anywhere near me."

> "I feel guilty, but the truth is, I am afraid of getting it from him. I do avoid any type of contact, sometimes even stuff I know is irrational like the same silverware or bottle of water. That sense of intimacy and trust is gone."

> "A definite relationship issue is transmission during sex. I feel it always affects us. He's afraid and I'm afraid; we're so uptight that it's not worth having a sex life anymore. Making love is supposed to be spontaneous and carefree. It's the opposite since his test came back positive."

> "The primary issue is the distance that's resulted because I'm afraid I'll pass it on to him, and though he doesn't like to admit it, he's afraid of it too. So we avoid talking about it and avoid doing anything that could put him in jeopardy."

Several narrative responses were congruent with recent medical advances in HIV/AIDS and the shifts in disease progression.

> "Honestly, it's just not that big a deal. If I get it, I get it. He's had it for years and is perfectly healthy. I'm willing to take that chance for us to get on with our lives together."

> "Fear of me getting the virus from him has lessened because we see how healthy he is. He's been positive for two years with not even a cold, so we started to be a little less overwhelmed about him transmitting it to me."

Another respondent expressed a recent controversial trend found among a small segment of those living with HIV called "bugchasing," when HIV-negative individuals purposely seek to contract HIV.

> "That he has it and I don't want it to keep us separate. I'm expecting to get it and in fact, hoping to so that whatever we go through, we go through together. Me being HIV positive will allow us to get on with our lives and not always be waiting for me to get it."

Case Studies

Case 1: Kevin and Anthony

Kevin is a thirty-three-year-old actor who comes from a large Irish family. He has been with his partner Anthony for six years. Anthony is an Italian man in his mid-thirties who is an accountant. Overall, their relationship has been relatively stable and both have been satisfied, but it has been injured by several significant conflicts around emotional and sexual intimacy. Through their six years together, they have weathered two near breakups. One conflict occurred when Kevin was not ready to commit to monogamy with Anthony after six months of dating. Kevin's reluctance was typical of previous relationships and would foreshadow an ongoing divide in this relationship. The second time of serious distress occurred two years into the relationship, due to Kevin's infidelity. After Anthony found out about the affair, the emotional repercussions included a break in trust on Anthony's part and Kevin felt that he was forever being punished for his infidelity.

Over the past four years, they have settled into a mutually satisfying relationship that has worked "pretty well most of the time." Then Kevin's HIV test came back positive. With this, the partners both experienced depression and anxiety. They drifted apart, and when they did talk, they fought.

They sought couple counseling, reporting that their relationship was deteriorating and they would like to save it if they could. After some initial history taking, the focus returned to the presenting problem.

KEVIN: I think all our old problems came back after the diagnosis and I don't think he can stand to be close to me.

THERAPIST: What makes you feel this way?

KEVIN: I get the feeling he's relieved not to make love anymore. I think he hasn't wanted to in a long time, and now he has an excuse. He doesn't want to get sick.

ANTHONY: Don't put this on me. What makes you think I'm relieved? That's how you feel maybe. I think you're not interested.

THERAPIST: Well, can each of you say how you really feel about this issue?

ANTHONY: I can. I can say that he's not interested and he's blaming me. He doesn't know how I feel. He's the one that's avoiding me.

KEVIN: This is why it turns into a fight. He's accusing me like it's my fault we don't have a sex life. I don't really know. I don't know how to get through to him.

THERAPIST: Let's see if, even for a minute, we can take the blame out of it and just describe what each of you experiences.

ANTHONY: I feel he's withdrawn from me. Sex is only one way. He's keeping his distance all-around and he makes it clear I should keep my distance too.

[Anthony's experience of Kevin's emotional distance is a distinct repeat of the preexisting dynamic within this dyad.]

THERAPIST: This sounds familiar to me. How has the HIV diagnosis brought this pattern up again?

KEVIN: Look. I'm kind of a loner. I always was. He knows I turn in when something upsets me, but he takes it personally when I'm quiet. I don't have the energy to pull him out or pull myself out to him. I'm hoping he'll be able to accept my need for space. I know he feels rejected, but I don't have the energy to pursue him right now.

ANTHONY: I can't always be expected to just withdraw, what about my needs? I also can't always be the one begging for attention. I give up.

THERAPIST: I hear that there is almost a sort of unspoken stand-off with each other; that you're both withdrawing from a certain level of intimacy. Kind of protecting yourselves. Any of that sound right?

This portion of the session reflects step 1 of emotionally focused couple therapy: assessment of their emotional and behavioral position patterns. In this phase of work, the therapist who is informed by EFT is simultaneously assessing and de-escalating a cycle of maladaptive patterns. This is done by interrupting the usual dynamic of mutual accusation and pointing out that they are experiencing similar emotions. As one partner accuses, the other accuses back and then withdraws. This results in both partners ultimately withdrawing and both partners inevitably feeling rejected. This problematic interaction pattern is identified and reflected to the partners. As the pattern is discussed, an interpretation is made regarding how this pattern maintains their attachment insecurities. The next excerpt of dialogue reflects step 2 of EFT: identifying and explaining the destructive interactional cycle.

THERAPIST: So there's been a pattern of mutual withdrawing that makes you both feel frustrated and insecure?

KEVIN: I guess I'm surprised to think of it that way. If I don't respond to him immediately, it's not that I don't want to be with him. It's more than I feel unsure. Things feel different. Like I said, he seems different.

THERAPIST: Different, how?

ANTHONY: Wait. I think I'm only different in response to you. I think you've backed away. But if you're going to be self-conscious, and make me feel self-conscious, I don't know how to be with you.

THERAPIST: And so, now it's not that much who started this distance. You can both see that certain behaviors maintain the distance and that's not really what either of you wants. Yet, it's important to wonder what purpose does the distance serve for each of you?

Understandably, high emotional reactivity exists on both parts, and Kevin and Anthony's emotional experiences are reflected back to them as they express their feelings both verbally and nonverbally. By asking them how they both feel about this issue, the emphasis is on identifying and expressing emotional experiences of each partner. This sets the stage for identifying emotions underlying the behaviors, as opposed to the "storyline" of the arguments: who did what to whom, etc.

Kevin and Anthony are helped to talk about how each feels easily rejected, tentative, and disoriented by the HIV diagnosis in their relationship. The HIV diagnosis did more than disorient this couple; it exacerbated preexisting issues around commitment and emotional intimacy that are now presenting in a lack of sexual and emotional intimacy. With some open-ended probing this couple is moved through step 3: facilitating discovery of unacknowledged feelings that have been fueled by the HIV diagnosis.

ANTHONY: I just feel the few times we've been together since the diagnosis, it's so awkward. It's different. It's like there's three of us in bed, me, you, and the virus. I can put it out of my mind at work and with some friends, but it's harder to put it out of my head when we're together.

KEVIN: Okay. Now we hear the truth. You think of me differently since the diagnosis. You *are* afraid of getting it! You're avoiding sex with me to avoid any chance of getting it. No wonder I feel rejected and no wonder I don't feel safe to be with you either.

THERAPIST: So neither of you feels emotionally safe with each other right now. What feels unsafe for each of you?

KEVIN: I feel like he's gonna reject me one way or another. If we don't have sex, he's gonna drift away, but I also feel like the little sex we've had since the diagnosis has been pretty disappointing. I know he was disappointed. I don't know that we can resurrect that part of our relationship. We couldn't really before the diagnosis. I don't think we know how to now.

ANTHONY: So you think that little of us? Of me? That I'm going somewhere because our sex life is stalled. That I would leave you? I can't believe you! I'll tell you what, if I leave, it'll be because all we do anymore is fight or avoid each other. Because you say things like that, that really hurt me . . . not because we're not having good sex. [Kevin is visibly frustrated and disgruntled by Anthony's comments.]

THERAPIST: Kevin, can you help Anthony understand your feelings better without accusing him?

KEVIN: I can try. I didn't mean to hurt you or say that the only thing we have going is our sex life. I was trying to say that that I worry that he's disappointed, and I guess I worry that if things don't improve, we'll just keep fighting and drifting . . . I feel him moving away.

ANTHONY: That's interesting. I feel like you left already. I feel like you're so busy expecting me to leave, that you left first.

As each partner described his emotional range of fear and anxiety regarding HIV transmission in their relationship, emotional experiences were elicited and full articulation was facilitated. Once their fears were expressed, Kevin and Anthony were asked to identify their own beliefs and behavioral patterns around the underlying threat to their attachment. For Kevin, his fear of infecting Anthony was fueled by his fear that Anthony would leave him because he had tested positive. Anthony was experiencing insecurity about Kevin's withdrawal. Further insight-oriented questions were used to help them more fully identify their unacknowledged feelings, and help them understand their conflict in terms of their unmet attachment needs (step 4).

THERAPIST: Does anything about this dynamic that you each need an emotional connection, but put up obstacles for fear of rejection, feel familiar from your families?

KEVIN: In a general way, sure. I could never really be myself or my family would reject me. I put off coming out because I knew they'd reject me. It was easier to be mad and distant with them than face that moment.

THERAPIST: Is it accurate to say, that one of the ways you have learned to protect yourself is to withdraw if you fear an emotional rejection?

KEVIN: I really only do this with people I'm close to. I don't do this dance if I don't care.

ANTHONY: So I guess I should feel honored.

THERAPIST: How *do* you feel?

ANTHONY: I know he's doing some of this to protect himself and I know his family has continued to reject him, but I'm not them and whatever magic he's doing to protect himself from me is backfiring.

THERAPIST: What would you say is familiar to you about how you've positioned yourself in this crisis?

ANTHONY: I guess much the same. Generally I become very internal when I think I might be hurt. I operated that way with my dad who was very unpredictable. I know if I don't feel safe, I tend to not have any expectations and pull into myself.

THERAPIST: One way of understanding your emotional experiences and behaviors, is that your withdrawal from one another actually points to how vulnerable you are to each other, how invested you truly [are] in one another's affections and interest. Does that make sense to you?

Kevin and Anthony were able to see the similar emotional issues with Kevin's family of origin—that Kevin feared coming out to his family would threaten his attachment to his family of origin and responded by withdrawing as he was doing with Anthony now. With some of this insight-oriented processing of the more latent material related to Kevin's feelings about attachment, the work always aimed to enhance Anthony's empathic understanding and emotional alliance with him.

As each partner was helped to express his emotional experiences, they both described a fear that if they pushed this issue by pursuing sex or sharing some of their fears about having sex, it might lead to a breakup. Helping Kevin and Anthony talk to each other about their respective anxieties about this issue, they came to realize that they shared the same underlying fear that HIV transmission, or acknowledgment of their fear of HIV transmission, could threaten their attachment. In this revelation, they shared a more complete empathic alliance. Through dyadic facilitation, Anthony was able to display his understanding to Kevin, and there was an increased empathic joining of each other's emotional experiences.

The second stage of the therapeutic intervention was aimed at restructuring the couple's emotional interaction and creating a more mutually conducive set of behavioral patterns. Because of their emotional conflict about attachment, maintaining or rejuvenating their sex life with HIV transmission while the virus was always lurking around the corner had become a "no-win" situation for both partners. After identifying how their behavioral positioning were informed by their underlying feelings, gentle suggestions were provided to enable them to soften these roles and allow for both to develop more constructive and affirming emotional patterns with each other that were based on their shared desire to stay together.

One example of steps 5-7 (promoting the owning of needs and of new/expanded aspects of the self and experience by the other; promoting acceptance of these aspects of self and experience by the other; facilitating the expression of needs and wants, and creating a safe emotional engagement) follows:

THERAPIST: Given that you are both feeling insecure and fearful of rejection with each other, what might be some of your real needs for each other at this time?

KEVIN: I suppose I need to know that he can talk about the HIV without freaking out, that he's not afraid of me or gonna leave at the drop of a hat.

ANTHONY: Drop of a hat? What's that supposed to mean? Afraid of you? Let me make this perfectly clear. I'm more freaked out by the thought that we could break up than the thought of getting HIV.

KEVIN: Well, okay. I didn't get that feeling from you, but okay. So could you not talk about us breaking up every time we have a fight, even sarcastically? It makes me feel like you're really thinking about it.

THERAPIST: How would you like to respond to Kevin's need, Anthony?

ANTHONY: I can try not to say stuff like that when we fight, but he has to stop saying that too, and stop egging me on to say it. It's not easy for me to hear when he says it either.

THERAPIST: Kevin, can you understand that Anthony is also left feeling upset and insecure when you threaten breaking up?

KEVIN: I guess. It's a little surprising to hear.

THERAPIST: It's surprising, but he says it upsets him also. Can you understand that he feels upset also?

KEVIN: I guess.

THERAPIST: How would you like to respond to his need for you not to jump to discussion of breaking up?

KEVIN: I guess to remember that it's just as upsetting to him as it is to me. I didn't know this.

THERAPIST: Can you both see that underneath the fights, there are similar feelings, and similar needs and wants about trying to stay together?

Although this was only one excerpt, many others fostered Kevin and Anthony's understanding of each other's needs and wants, as well as promoting mutual acceptance of each other's needs concerning the issues raised by fear of HIV transmission. Each was helped to understand how his fear of HIV transmission heightened his anxiety about the couple's attachment and heightened the need for reassurance about their commitment to each other.

Steps 8 and 9 emphasize the building and consolidation of more adaptive interactional positioning and behaviors. With Kevin and Anthony, this included discussion of how they could respond to each other's needs.

THERAPIST: It seems that a feeling of insecurity and fear of rejection is swirling around both of you since the HIV diagnosis. It may come out in somewhat different ways, but both of you have identified that your instinct is to withdraw to avoid feeling rejected. Your dance of self-protection has left both of you feeling alone and insecure. What could you do differently to take care of each other and the relationship more satisfactorily?

KEVIN: Well, if we can keep our emotions more under control, it sounds like it would be helpful to avoid threatening to break up when we fight, even sarcastically.

ANTHONY: It would be helpful to be more direct and more attentive so neither of us feels rejected. I didn't realize he felt as bad as I did.

KEVIN: [Laughing] Great! We've both felt lousy. I know this . . . whoever initiates intimacy of any kind gets a gold star and I guess just has to leave it to faith that he won't be rejected.

ANTHONY: [Sarcastically, but in good humor] He?

In this last excerpt, the reader can see not only the consolidation of new behavioral and emotional positioning but the application of the three practice principles central to ICT. Each partner was helped to identify targeted behaviors in the other that he wished could be altered. Each partner was also helped to move toward acceptance of the emotional experiences and needs of his mate, and in the last exchange, when the partners are asked how could they take better care of their relationship, unified detachment was employed. With such a question, we externalize the problematic issue, so that the problem is not all Kevin's or all Anthony's, but reframed as a shared problem of how to make the relationship safer for each of them. This reframing was used to help them resolve some of their preexisting issues that were related to intimacy, commitment, and basic trust. They emerged from therapy better able to develop the types of emotional expressions and positions that revitalized their emotional and physical intimacy as they no longer viewed the issue of transmission as an injury to their attachment to each other, but in fact as an opportunity to cement their devotion.

This is a somewhat simplified overview of a therapeutic process with a complicated issue that may affect couples quite differently, but the underlying feelings both partners experienced, HIV transmission as a threat to their attachment, is of critical importance. For the couple practitioner working with this issue it is key to foster and facilitate a safe atmosphere so that each partner can be forthcoming about his or her fears and anxieties regarding HIV transmission. Sometimes therapy may remain on the manifest level, and sometimes it may help the couple move toward the latent regarding their issues of attachment.

The therapist work from an emotionally oriented approach aims to unearth emotional experiences that activate partners' core beliefs about themselves. After eliciting these feeling states and belief systems, the therapist facilitates a new emotional experience between partners that has shifted with deeper understanding and acceptance of each other's emotional sensitivities around their attachment. The partners will then be helped to organize more adaptive emotional positions in relation to each other. Thus the work is done in two stages: eliciting the core emotional experiences and then restructuring the more empathetically attuned emotional positions in relation to each other.

The impact of fear of HIV transmission has been documented as a primary issue and has been described by respondents and illustrated in more depth by our case study. Although fear of HIV transmission between discordant partners might appear to be an expected stressor, it may affect different couples in many different ways. The following cases will be presented in summary to add a different dimension to this issue.

Case II: Angela and Rick

Angela is a twenty-nine-year-old Hispanic woman who has been living with her boyfriend Rick for five years. They share a history of substance abuse and alcoholism, and both have been clean and sober for nearly the five years that they have been together. Angela was diagnosed with HIV three years ago. Rick, aged forty, gets tested every six months and has remained HIV negative. Angela has experienced HIV-related illness that required hospitalization. She has been treated effectively with combination therapy since this episode two years ago. This was a traumatic event for each of them individually and as a couple. Their relationship has many strengths and appears to be based on an authentic acceptance of each other, but they have not been able to reestablish an intimate relationship since Angela's hospitalization. They have difficulty talking to each other honestly about the impact of HIV in their lives.

Following the emotionally focused couple therapy framework, the first stage of work with this couple was to assess their emotional and behavioral patterns that had been activated by the events surrounding Angela's HIV diagnosis and hospitalization. Open-ended questions facilitated their respective feeling states in the therapeutic encounter with an aim to rejuvenate their empathic connection and attachment to each other.

Angela's HIV diagnosis and hospitalizations were thoroughly unexpected and catalyzed a centripetal response in which both partners reported feeling closer to each other than ever. However, after each crisis, further distance ensued in their emotional and intimate lives together. They have had difficulty maintaining a satisfactory sex life as well as talking about how Angela's health status made them both feel. Angela was fearful that she could infect Rick. She tried to protect him from her fears and anxieties about the potential of her illness and in order to physically protect him, her behavior has been one of disinterest and strident independence. When he has shown interest in her sexually or concern for her overall well-being, she backs off, and then he backs off as well. When he is too disengaged for her level of comfort though, she pursues him. Rick is confused and feels that Angela has been giving him mixed messages. He feels Angela has not been interested in intimacy and that he should conform to her needs, but when he does pull away, she changes her mind and wants to be close with him. His behavior has been very caring and overprotective, but lately has become unpredictable.

In unearthing some of Angela and Rick's core emotional experiences about relationships, Angela was able to provide relevant history. Angela's sibling subsystem plays a critical role in her current feelings and behaviors with Rick concerning her HIV status. Angela is the only female in her family of origin and is the youngest of five. Reflecting on her childhood emotional states, she described her parents as physically and emotionally unavailable. Her brothers were her primary attachment, and her relationship with her two eldest brothers was the most adaptive but still unpredictable.

Her brothers were approving of Angela when she evidenced self-sufficient behaviors. She reports that any expression of emotional dependence was met with disapproval and even ridicule. When she was physically ill or emotionally frightened, her brothers were emotionally unavailable and the ridicule or chastising she received made her feel guilty. This dynamic and her interpretation of it served as an emotional blueprint for adult attachments. Her attachment style with adults seemed to be marked by ambivalence. She desired an emotional intimacy, but was also fearful of truly allowing herself to become dependent. The more dependent she authentically felt, the more depressed she became. For her, this dependency was a sign of weakness and she feared it would drive Rick away. This core emotional experience and belief about herself manifested in behavioral patterns that can be characterized as ambivalent. Her cues seemed to inevitably push her partner away when she wished for closeness the most. This dynamic unfolded with Rick after the HIV diagnosis and then again after the hospitalization.

For Rick, his reaction was that Angela was self-sufficient and preferred not to engage in any intimacy or any potentially upsetting discussions about HIV. Rick was the youngest of three in a single parent family. He describes his mother as depressed and alcoholic and explains that his mother was unavailable to all of them, particularly Rick whose father left her after Rick was born. Rick described an avoidant attachment style with his mother. He also explained that he felt responsible for his mother's depression. In his adult relationships with women, he consistently engaged with depressed women who were disparaging toward him. He often felt responsible for his partner's depression. With Angela, he had his most adaptive partnership in which Angela was somewhat depressed, but had the capacity for joy and intermittent intimacy. Following her HIV diagnosis and hospitalization, Angela became more depressed. In response, Rick felt responsible for her depression and her misfortune. They had both used drugs together, but he had not contracted the virus and she did.

He feared she was mad at him and she was withdrawing more out of anger than sadness.

Symmetrically, they both withdrew, avoiding further attachment injury. The circular causality ensued—the more depressed she became, the more he withdrew and the more he withdrew, the more depressed she became. By the time they approached counseling, they were both depressed and isolated from one another.

ANGELA: I just feel dead. I have no feeling. I don't want to upset him, but I don't think he should be near me when I'm like this.

THERAPIST: Why?

ANGELA: I don't want him to be burdened by me. I don't want him to get sick.

RICK: This is how she talks. I don't know what I'm supposed to do. I want to take care of her, but she won't let me. I'm not afraid of seeing her upset, and I know how to keep myself safe.

THERAPIST: So Angela, you're worried that your feelings are too much for Rick to carry? And Rick you're feeling frustrated because you'd like to be more supportive of her? Angela, can you tell us more what it is you worry about, about Rick?

ANGELA: I think it would be best for him to keep his distance. I worry, what if they're wrong and he could get the HIV from shared towels or kitchenware, or kissing? I just don't want him to be affected at all. It's my problem. I can take care of this myself. [She starts crying.] He's such a good guy. I don't want to burden him.

RICK: How can you say that? How can you possibly say that? I don't want anything else. I'm not afraid of seeing you upset and I'm not afraid of getting sick. [Turning to therapist,] I think this is her problem. I've never said or done anything, but try and help her.

After eliciting some of these emotional experiences, Angela and Rick were helped to better understand and accept each other's current emotional experiences of each other and how this has been intensified by Angela's HIV diagnosis. Rick was able to understand that any feelings of dependency Angela experienced had an ominous undertow that resulted in her efforts toward self-sufficiency and independence. As Rick came forward to take care of Angela, she was frightened of the dependency she felt with him. She pulled away seemingly more depressed, and this made Rick feel responsible for her depression and incapable of relieving her sadness. Insight-oriented questions on how they have experienced their previous relationship dynamics that were similar and emphasized how their underlying feelings about themselves and their respective attachment seemed to guide this current dynamic.

Therapy also included identifying those respective behaviors that needed to shift as they created confusion or unwanted reactions, such as Angela drawing away from Rick. Again, the tool of unified detachment was used successfully. How can they share the responsibility for improving this dynamic instead of blaming or accusing each other? They were helped to develop a pattern that encouraged Angela to trust Rick when she felt dependent and helped Rick to depersonalize Angela's depression. Therapy concluded with the identification of more empathic and adaptive interactional patterns that interrupted the circular causality and turned their behaviors and their reactions to a more positive pattern. The more he pursued her attentively, the less depressed she became in regard to him. Although they certainly continued to cope with stressors related to HIV transmission, their communication and behavioral patterns significantly enhanced their emotional satisfaction with each other.

Case III: Ray and Michael

Ray and Michael are both in their early forties. Ray is African American and Michael is Jewish/Italian. They have been together for seven years. Michael tested positive seven years ago during a routine examination. Ray was tested shortly after and tested negative. They never spoke about the source of HIV transmission. Michael has not experienced any HIV-related illness. Initially, he avoided medication treatment. As his viral load became higher several years ago, he tried several versions of combination therapy. He was not able to tolerate the side effects and returned to alternative treatments that have been largely effective. In the past year, they have been fighting more often and more intensely. They both describe trouble in the relationship stemming from "old issues" as well as the HIV. Michael avoided any discussion of potential illness or HIV transmission. Ray felt anxious and unsettled about Michael's health, HIV transmission between them, and fear about Michael's inability to tolerate combination therapies. Ray tried to initiate safer sex practices, different sexual activities than engaged in prior to the diagnosis, but Michael was resistant. After some experimentation with sex practices that were safer but "less satisfying" in Ray's words, he gave up. This couple exhibited the classic "pursuer-distancer" dynamic around issues of sexual intimacy. As Ray became anxious to discuss safer sex issues, Michael withdrew more. The more that Michael experienced Ray "coming after me to talk about HIV" the more he avoided any quality time or sexual time with Ray as this made him extremely anxious and self-conscious about his HIV status. This pattern intensified with Ray pursuing Michael and Michael running away from emotional or physical intimacy to ward off talking about HIV.

Initial therapeutic stages consisted of eliciting Ray and Michael's emotional experiences and interactional behavioral patterns. Assessment of their current emotional experiences and their respective mutual needs and wants as a couple was a lengthy and complex undertaking with Ray and Michael. There was great conflict with each other, within each of them, and with the therapeutic process itself. To provide a safe atmosphere and facilitate authentic communications about honest feelings, Ray, and particularly Michael, required variation in therapeutic approaches.

In addition to EFCT and ICT, this couple responded well to the use of some cognitive interventions as well. Michael was unable to identify his emotional experiences, needs, and wants, and had difficulty relating to Ray's expressed emotional experiences. With each attempt, Michael felt more hopeless and Ray became more frustrated. We moved away from the emotional plane and shifted toward their cognitive processes concerning each other and this issue. As Dattilio and Bevilacqua (2000) explain, this does not mean that the sole focus was cognitive, but rather that in addition to emotion and behavior, cognitive patterns are also addressed. The relationship between the cognitive, affect, and then behavioral patterns was a more holistic approach that was a better match for this particular couple. Starting with their respective thought patterns about how HIV has affected their relationship was an easier task for both partners. With dyadic facilitation, they were able to identify the thought patterns that led to this mutually unsatisfying pursuer-distancer dynamic.

In session and in response to journal entries, those thoughts that were based in distortion on the part of both partners were identified and challenged. When Michael hears Ray express fear or anxiety about HIV transmission, Michael's automatic thought is, "He sees me only as my HIV now." This is an example of dichotomous or polarized thinking, which refers to those thoughts one has that are "all or nothing." In addition to dichotomous thinking, Michael also evidenced mindreading patterns. He often assumed he knew what was going through his partner's mind. For example, "What Ray really thinks is. . . ." Michael thought that underneath all their fights, Ray was terrified of getting AIDS (though they never had this conversation). Whether this was true or not in reality, it was what was informing Michael's behavior. The following excerpt illustrates a pivotal component of their dynamic.

THERAPIST: So you assume Ray is terrified. We don't know for sure whether he is or isn't, but how does Ray's perceived "state of terror" make you feel?

MICHAEL: Like I'm living with my mother. He's all over me. Everything I do he's afraid is unhealthy for me or for him.

THERAPIST: And how does it make you behave?

MICHAEL: It makes me avoid him like the damn plague!

This portion of the work focused on how Michael positioned himself based on his assumptions. When Ray was brought into correct Michael's mind reading, an important shift happened.

RAY: Well I'm not terrified and I don't behave as if I'm terrified. I'm more concerned than anything else. I'm concerned for your health and I'm concerned about our life together. Can't I feel that way without you being so repulsed?

THERAPIST: What did you hear Ray say to you?

MICHAEL: That he's not terrified of AIDS. He's lying though. I don't believe him! He won't tell the truth!

RAY: Well, what am I supposed to do about that? He's impossible. Screw you already! Don't believe me then!

Often, with each step forward, one or both sabotaged any progress made in their relationship as seen in the previous dialogue. A worker can enter into this angry moment with many different interventions. One choice could be silence, allowing the couple to naturally try to repair the damage. One could follow a cognitive approach and pursue what types of thought patterns preceded this type of angry exchange, such as what were you thinking that made you feel so angry with Michael? Cognitive therapy would try to identify those thoughts that might be irrational or distorted, resulting in an intense emotional reaction. As the connection between thought patterns and emotional experiences are tested and reality checked, partners can be helped to restructure those thoughts that are detrimental to the relationship.

If you are working from an integrative couples approach you could choose to point out that this miscommunication and mistrust is a problem both Michael and Ray share and need to address. The emotionally focused approach would try to delve into the underlying feelings of Michael and Ray that resulted in these behavioral positions. One could try all of these approaches and others and still not be able to soothe the anger and hurt in the room.

Emotionally focused therapy was the approach of choice in this moment because this exchange was rife with affect, both primary (those that precede the angry outburst, commonly hurt) and secondary (lashing-out comments) for both partners.

THERAPIST: It's clear you're both very angry right now. You may be too angry to try and understand what the other is feeling. Even though you're both really frustrated and mad, can either of you reach out in any way to try and explain what you felt that made you lash out? [This is referred to as the gauntlet challenge, an intervention in which the couple is challenged to break out of their interdependent standoff.]

RAY: I don't think I can say anything. It doesn't matter what I say if he doesn't believe me. I think this one's up to him to fix.

MICHAEL: Look, I don't want to fight. I'm just saying you are really, really scared that I may get sick. I think you're really, really scared that you could get the virus. Can't you just fess up to that and not gaslight me?

THERAPIST: Listen, Michael. Let me ask you, what is it you felt when he said he wasn't terrified?

MICHAEL: I felt . . . it's weird . . . felt betrayed. I felt like hurt that he felt he can't tell me the truth . . . that he's afraid it would hurt me to admit it.

THERAPIST: Ok. That's how you felt before you felt angry. Ray, you don't have to agree with his take on this, you maybe can't even understand it, but can you relate to his feeling hurt?

RAY: I guess. I don't even know anymore. I don't want to fight either, but look at what he's doing. He's putting me in a no-win. If I tell him I'm terrified then I'm a big worry wart. If I tell him I'm not, then I'm a liar.

THERAPIST: So you feel pretty frustrated right now?

RAY: Uh-huh.

THERAPIST: Underneath your retaliation to him was a sense of despair?

RAY: Exactly. I give up.

THERAPIST: Now it's your turn, Michael. When you see that Ray feels so frustrated, can you get what he's going through?

MICHAEL: Of course. I'm frustrated also and I don't want to drive him crazy. I just wish he'd back off a bit. Is that so terrible?

Therapy shifted to further exploration of underlying feelings about their relationship and their respective and mutual attachment needs and wants. With each disruption in empathic joining, Michael and Ray were helped to understand how their distortions in thoughts fed the dynamics that interrupted their sustained emotional intimacy. They worked on understanding what purpose was served by avoiding intimacy. A long-standing issue for Ray was his struggle with depression and low self-esteem. Though he has often feared being alone, he has also taken some comfort in being with a partner who does not demand much emotional intimacy from him. Michael's recent distancing provoked further depression, but also a familiar pattern in which he was the arbiter of the level of intimacy in his relationships. In addition, he has had a very low libido and was relieved that Michael made no demands on him for sex.

For Michael, he avoided all discussion of HIV, but this was consistent with his earlier avoidance of anything emotionally difficult between himself and Ray and previous partners. He has always been very internal and very self-sufficient, and Ray's need for intimacy was perceived as a signal of crisis due to his diagnosis.

With each new awareness of how the HIV diagnosis exacerbated their preexisting issues (individually and as a dyad) came more motivation and capacity to shift their dyadic behaviors to a more positive pattern. There was always a need to strengthen their empathic connection to each other. Although they certainly continued to cope with stressors related and unrelated to HIV transmission, the diminution of cognitive distortions, improved communication, and deeper empathic connection stabilized their attachment to each other significantly.

SUMMARY

Couples facing any chronic or potentially terminal illness must negotiate numerous emotional challenges within the relationship. This chapter has identified an emotional challenge unique to HIV/AIDS: fear of HIV transmission. This research has indicated that anxieties about HIV transmission with couples of mixed HIV status are common, regardless of sexual orientation and ethnicity, and may be somewhat more prevalent in heterosexual relationships than in gay male relationships. The narrative responses illustrate the range of ways a couple may feel impacted by this issue, and the case presentations provide further insight into how couples may cope with this dynamic. Practitioners treating couples of mixed HIV status should anticipate that this issue may be present and should assess whether it has presented any particular challenges to the security of the relationship. As evidenced in case presentations, different theoretical frameworks may be applied, but certainly EFCT can be a primary approach in one's repertoire. The critical concepts of EFCT, such as attachment needs, the underlying emotional experiences of respective partners, interactional dynamics, and the primary goal of improving an empathic alliance between partners, can be used quite effectively to inform clinical practice with couples of mixed HIV status facing issues around HIV transmission in their relationship.

Chapter 7

Shifts in Emotional Intimacy

"We were never as close as the day I was diagnosed. Now we drift along until each doctor's appointment and then we're really close again."

OVERVIEW

Many dyadic emotional shifts, some profound, some more superficial and seemingly temporary, were identified as a result of one partner's positive HIV status. Emotional intimacy may mean something different to each individual respondent and each couple. From open-ended responses and cases, intimacy generally referred to feelings of closeness, positive attachment, and feeling understood and accepted by each other.

For many, the HIV diagnosis opened up a deeper level of attachment and intimacy. Feeling that their time together as a couple, a healthy couple, may be in jeopardy, they have experienced an increase in intimacy and have valued their commitment to each other more. For others, the diagnosis and the difference in HIV status evoked obstacles to sustained emotional intimacy between partners. For other couples, the HIV diagnosis brought more emotional distance, with one or both partners recoiling due to depression or anxiety. The narrative responses demonstrated that there were also couples who experienced fluctuating emotional intimacy, feeling closer around the issues of the diagnosis and shared fears of illness, yet more distance caused by feelings of depression, betrayal, or withdrawal from each other. However the HIV diagnosis affected a couple's emotional intimacy, it is evident that the intimate lives of a couple are deeply impacted. The range and trends of how a couple's dynamics can and have been shifted by HIV will be identified and clarified in this chapter.

QUANTITATIVE FINDINGS

When HIV serostatus is analyzed, one finds that the changes in emotional intimacy are experienced equally by those who were diagnosed, as well as by their partners. This confirms that both partners experience shifts in intimacy regardless of which partner is HIV positive or HIV negative. This concurs with relevant literature on the subject (Adam and Sears, 1996; Chidwick and Borrill, 1996; Hoffman, 1996; Klimes et al., 1992; Williams-Saporito, 1998).

Interestingly, couples who identify themselves as heterosexual report more changes in their emotional intimacy as a result of HIV than do gay couples (Table 7.1). Nearly 100 percent of heterosexual couples strongly agreed that there were shifts in emotional intimacy, whereas only 50 percent of gay couples strongly agreed. This supports relevant research that finds that women in heterosexual serodiscordant relationships are more likely to react to an HIV diagnosis with depressive reactions that would surely affect their ability to maintain emotional intimacy with their partners (Lambiase et al., 1994; Mayer and Wells, 1997; Van der Straten et al., 1998). In addition, women are reported to withdraw from emotional confrontations with their male partners more often than men when depressed (Van der Straten et al., 1998) (Table 7.2). Therefore, one can understand that heterosexual couples of mixed HIV status may be more vulnerable to emotional shifts in their relationships. Another interesting pat-

TABLE 7.1. Sexual orientation: Shifts in emotional intimacy are of primary concern.

	Strongly agree	Agree	Disagree	Strongly disagree	Total
Heterosexual	38 (95%)	0	2 (5%)	0	40
Homosexual	24 (50%)	18 (37.5%)	6 (12.5%)	0	48
Total	62	18	8	0	88

TABLE 7.2. Gender in heterosexual relationships: Shifts in emotional intimacy are of primary concern.

	Strongly agree	Agree	Disagree	Strongly disagree	Total
Female	13 (65%)	7 (35%)		0	20
Male	49 (72%)	11 (16%)	8 (12%)	0	68
Total	62	18	8	0	88

tern emerged from narrative responses and cases. It seems HIV diagnosis in heterosexual couples tended to create more shifts and emotional distancing, whereas the HIV diagnosis in gay relationships tended to create more emotional intimacy (Huggins et al., 1991).

A noteworthy phenomenon that supports the wish and effort toward intimacy in the gay male community is the purposeful attempts of HIV-negative individuals to become HIV positive. This may be an effort to master the uncertainty of HIV contraction, a political statement, a result of mental and emotional exhaustion about safer sex prevention, or a characterological depression or suicidal tendency (Yep, Lovaas, and Pagonis, 2002). Within the context of a committed relationship, there is a conscious effort of pursuing HIV transmission so that the partners are not physically or psychologically separated by serostatus. The intrapsychic and interpersonal dynamics will be further discussed in detail in the case studies presented in this chapter.

There did not appear to be any noteworthy differences in how emotional intimacy is affected by one partner's positive HIV status across different ethnic backgrounds. Table 7.3 indicates that, in general, the majority of respondents from all ethnicities reported shifts in their emotional intimacy as a result of their mixed HIV status.

A greater majority of the female respondents (85 percent) than the male respondents (66 percent) reported shifts in emotional intimacy. This finding concurs with the earlier findings regarding sexual orientation, in which women tend to either experience and/or report emotional shifts as a partner in a serodiscordant relationship more often than men, and that heterosexual partners coping with serodiscordance may experience more emotional instability than gay male relationships.

Based on twenty heterosexual couples, when the female is HIV positive she experiences more emotional shifts with her partner than the converse (Table 7.4). Although HIV-positive men do report emotional shifts in their relationship due to their own HIV-positive status, they are more deeply affected when they are HIV negative and their partner is HIV positive (Table 7.5). Though a small trend, it is still in-

TABLE 7.3. Ethnicity: Shifts in emotional intimacy are of primary concern.

	Strongly agree	Agree	Disagree	Strongly disagree	Total
African American	13 (57%)	7 (30%)	3 (13%)	0	23
Hispanic	19 (68%)	6 (21%)	3 (11%)	0	28
White	30 (81%)	5 (14%)	2 (5%)	0	37
Total	62	18	8	0	88

TABLE 7.4. HIV-positive partners in heterosexual relationships: Shifts in emotional intimacy are of primary concern.

	Strongly agree	Agree	Disagree	Strongly disagree	Total
HIV-positive women	2 (20%)	6 (60%)	2 (20%)	0	10
HIV-positive men	6 (60%)	1 (10%)	2 (20%)	1 (10%)	10
HIV-negative women	8 (80%)	2 (20%)	0	0	10
HIV-negative men	3 (30%)	3 (30%)	3 (30%)	1 (10%)	10
Total	19	12	7	2	40

teresting to consider the cultural gender stereotypes and how they may contribute to men feeling the impact in their emotional relationship more when their female partner tests positive than when they test positive.

Another variable affecting shifts in emotional intimacy in couples of mixed HIV status is how long the partners have been together (Table 7.6). For those that have been together for more than five years, the shifts in emotional intimacy were less than those who have been together for less than five years. This was an expected outcome as often the longer the couple is together, the more effective their coping skills for crisis that may upset the stability of the relationship (Jacobsen and Christensen, 1996a).

As one might anticipate, those couples who entered their courtship aware of the presence of HIV experienced significantly fewer emo-

TABLE 7.5. Serostatus: Shifts in emotional intimacy are of primary concern.

	Strongly agree	Agree	Disagree	Strongly disagree	Total
HIV positive	31 (70.5%)	9 (20.5%)	4 (9%)	0	44
HIV negative	31 (70.5%)	9 (20.5%)	4 (9%)	0	44
Total	62	18	8	0	88

TABLE 7.6. Length of relationship: Shifts in emotional intimacy are of primary concern.

	Strongly agree	Agree	Disagree	Strongly disagree	Total
Less than 5 years	32 (84%)	6 (16%)	0	0	38
More than 5 years	30 (60%)	12 (24%)	8 (16%)	0	50
Total	62	18	8	0	88

tional changes in the relationship than those who learned of the HIV diagnosis during the relationship (Table 7.7). Only 31 percent of those who knew of the diagnosis beforehand experienced shifts in emotional intimacy as a result of the HIV diagnosis, whereas 93 percent of those who found out about the HIV after the relationship started experienced emotional shifts in the relationship.

Perhaps the most dramatic finding in this area is that those couples who have experienced any HIV-related illness have been twice as likely to report emotional shifts in the relationship as those couples who have not (Table 7.8). The emotional experience of an HIV-related illness, even one that is managed quickly and without any serious medical setbacks, provokes an understandably profound emo-

TABLE 7.7. When couple learned of HIV diagnosis: Shifts in emotional intimacy are of primary concern.

	Strongly agree	Agree	Disagree	Strongly disagree	Total
Diagnosed before relationship	10 (31%)	14 (44%)	8 (25%)	0	32
Diagnosed in relationship	52 (93%)	4 (7%)	0	0	56
Total	62	18	8	0	88

TABLE 7.8. HIV-related illness: Shifts in emotional intimacy are of primary concern.

	Strongly agree	Agree	Disagree	Strongly disagree	Total
Have had HIV illness	38 (79%)	9 (19%)	1 (2%)	0	48
Have not had HIV illness	24 (60%)	9 (22.5%)	7 (17.5%)	0	40
Total	62	18	8	0	88

tional reaction in each individual and within the relationship. As each partner deals with emotional reactions, the relationship may experience increased closeness concerning some issues and increased distance regarding other issues. This can be understood as an expectable dynamic with any illness in a relationship, but the uniqueness of HIV is illustrated in the narrative comments that follow.

QUALITATIVE FINDINGS

Narrative Responses to Open-Ended Questions

This section includes excerpts from the respondents' open-ended responses. It is organized according to certain trends and patterns that emerged from their own experiences. The three trends included an increase in emotional intimacy, emotional distancing, and a fluctuation between emotional intimacy and distancing as a result of mixed HIV status in the relationship.

Increase in Emotional Intimacy

Due to both illness and potentially less time together, many said they related with greater honesty, trust, and value. This was highlighted with consistent and touching poignancy:

> "We are more dear to each other because after the positive test, we understand the fragility of our life together."

> "HIV makes me realize how much I love him, how concerned I am for him and how much I want him to know I'll be with him."

> "The crisis of him being positive really brought us together."

> "She thought I'd leave when she tested positive, when I stayed, that's when we really became a couple."

> "I'm healthy now, but who knows when something might happen. I think it makes us feel closer that we both know our time together may look very different at any time."

> "I think it helps us to work together and not fight about the small day-to-day stuff as much as we might."

Increase in Emotional Distancing

The difference in HIV status created emotional distance of varying forms as expressed by respondents:

> "Since he tested HIV, I can never trust him again. I can never feel close to him again."

A husband wrote about his HIV positive wife,

> "I always worry that if I tell her how I really feel, it'll just upset her more. I think we both have drifted trying to protect each other."

Emotional Distance Due to Protecting Each Other

> "In a way, we've drifted because I don't want to upset her with anything. So I don't really tell her when I worry about her health or our future."

> "I don't want to bring up anything that would cause him stress. I keep my problems to myself now because what I go through seems so unimportant. The main thing is just to keep his stress level low."

> "I know we should talk about more serious things about his HIV, what if he gets sick, but I guess we [would] both rather avoid it. In a way, it's like there's a secret between us that we both know about, but it still kind of divides us."

Fluctuations in Emotional Intimacy

Some couples simultaneously pull toward each other to feel close during an emotional crisis and push away to defend against their feelings about loss or anxiety. Minuchin (1984), Bowen (1978), and other leaders in family therapies have referred to this as the inevitable centrifugal forces (those which pull partners apart) and centripetal forces (those which push partners closer) that occur in families and couples at developmental milestones or emotional crises. Further, within each individual there is often a conscious and/or unconscious process with these conflicting pulls. One instinct propels the individual toward his or her mate in the primary attachment whereas another instinct may tell him or her to withdraw from the mate. In the case of physical illness, it is not uncommon to see a partner regress and withdraw to either "lick his or her wounds alone" or even return to family of origin for soothing and comfort he or she knows and trusts from an earlier time. Examples of such dynamics are provided by the respondents:

> "It's funny. We're both closer and further since the HIV diagnosis. It depends when you catch us."

> "In some ways, particularly around his health we're much closer, but in other ways, about our sex life and day-to-day stuff, I miss him."

> "We're so much closer, but it's hard to sustain because there is a part of me that doesn't want to stay this close with him. I don't want to be this vulnerable with him."

> "I'd say we're more distant overall, avoiding heart-to-heart talks, but in certain moments when we do talk about my illness, I feel closer to him than before I was ill."

Case Studies

Case I: Increase in Emotional Intimacy Due to Protecting Each Other: Rob and John

Rob is a twenty-eight-year-old Jewish male. He is from upstate New York where he is the younger of two sons. His parents were described as "exhausted and depressed." Rob has had a conflictual and insecure relationship with his family of origin, marked by a distant formality. Although his family knows he is gay, they do not know that he tested HIV positive two years ago. Rob describes a long history of dysthymia. He is quiet, somewhat antisocial, and has difficulty identifying and articulating his emotional experiences. He has recently been on antidepressants that have lifted his spirits enough to "work" on his relationship with John, his partner of two years.

John is a thirty-eight-year-old Jewish-Italian male. He is an actor who comes from a large family in which he is the oldest son. He describes his family as "loud" and "emotionally abusive." He has suffered periodically from depression and anxiety around traveling and being separated from Rob for any lengthy period of time.

This closeness has sustained them through several ongoing conflicts about money and friends, but they have been fighting more and more about day-to-day issues since Rob's HIV diagnosis six months ago.

Rob and John came into couple counseling trying to find tools to ease the day-to-day fighting and learn how to talk about the "big issues" between them, such as money, friends, and their difference in HIV status, without fighting. They presented as particularly motivated and emotionally allied to work on these issues.

Rob and John did not need to be empathetically joined with each other. Through opening sessions, it was clear that Rob and John shared a complementary and supportive relationship marked by a stable emotional intimacy. Both partners had experienced stigma and rejection as gay men and found solace in each other against their perceived enemies. This relationship has served Rob and John as a safe haven from the rejection and conflict they each experienced in their family of origin. This safe haven, however, did not allow for differentiation; new friends and interests of either partner were often experienced by both as a potential threat to the security of their bond. When either partner shifted this unspoken contract, high anxiety resulted. The potential hazard with this level of enmeshment was that neither was able to individuate. The diagnosis of HIV was the first injury to this merged state they created.

With Rob's HIV diagnosis, each partner's preexisting emotional states of depression intensified. As each partner saw his mate struggling emotionally, he took on overprotective stances with the other. As they chose not to share their anxieties and sadness about the diagnosis with one another (to protect each other, and maybe themselves), Rob and John began to fight more about superficial day-to-day issues.

ROB: I just feel like we never regrouped after my diagnosis. We've been fighting about stupid things and just not getting along.

JOHN: I really don't know what happened. But he's right. We're just fighting and it's the last thing I want. Our fighting doesn't get us anywhere and I don't want to upset him.

THERAPIST: Tell me a little about how the relationship feels different since the diagnosis.

JOHN: We never use[d] to fight. We really see things very much the same and have always gotten along really well. The one or two areas of conflict we might have had we were able to resolve. Or at least I thought we were. I want to be of support to him through this. I try, but he won't let me take care of him. I actually feel like we've drifted since the diagnosis.

THERAPIST: So in some ways, since the diagnosis your intent is to be supportive and reduce stress for Rob, yet you find the two of you are fighting more and feeling more distant? Rob, how about you?

ROB: I have no idea. We've always been so close. Our friends are all jealous of how happy we are. I feel like I can't talk to him about the diagnosis.

THERAPIST: Why? What makes you feel you can't talk to him about it?

ROB: It makes me so sad to see him upset. I don't want to upset him.

THERAPIST: A part of you would like to protect him from feeling upset, and a part of you might want to avoid feeling sad? Sometimes it's hard to really share with your partner, because that involves really feeling whatever you've been going through.

JOHN: Yeah. Any time we do really try to talk about it, he becomes very sad. I think both of us are avoiding it to protect each other, but maybe to protect ourselves also. I guess it's easier to fight about the dishes than this. I guess we've been pretty busy avoiding this.

This is one brief excerpt after several sessions aimed to uncover how Rob and John's underlying anxiety about the HIV diagnosis was displaced onto less provocative content. In addition, this dynamic fostered an emotional distance because intimacy was too threatening given their respective level of upset by the potential hazard HIV might pose to their bond.

Emotionally focused treatment reflected the positioning each had taken on and the underlying emotions that fueled these positions. With these reflections, the couple's fighting diminished and the couple was readied to own their own emotional needs before they tried to take care of each other's assumed emotional needs. Once the partners owned their individual disowned emotions, they were more able to develop emotional responses that were more finely attuned to their distinct emotional experiences and needs in the face of the HIV diagnosis. The day-to-day fighting served the purpose of deflecting or masking their underlying feelings of anxiety evoked by the HIV diagnosis.

Case II: Fluctuations in Emotional Intimacy: Mike and Claude

Mike and Claude are a couple who sought counseling in response to increased fighting about many issues, including their difference in HIV status. Mike is a thirty-year-old Italian-Portugese lawyer. He is from a large, lower-middle-class family in which he is one of five children. He has had a difficult time coming out as a gay man to his family. The process started in his late teens as he began to tell one sibling at a time. Initially, each sibling had mixed reactions at best. Although his brothers and sisters came to fully accept him, his relationship with his mother has remained conflictual and strained. His dad passed away several years ago. Mike is successful in his career and enjoys an active social life with old friends as well as recently established friends. He has no history of depression or anxiety, but he has struggled periodically with anger management.

Claude is a twenty-nine-year-old African American. He is a physical education instructor in a public school. He has one younger sister who has a range of serious medical disabilities. Claude was raised by his mother and was a caretaker for both his mother and sister. His mother suffered from depression and alcoholism. His sister required assistance with most physical activities. He remains very involved and very close with his mother and sister who live near him.

Mike and Claude met each other in a summer project in their neighborhood when they were teens. They continued their friendship through college. Although not romantically involved with each other, they built a close friendship as they came out to each other in their early twenties. They both dated other men and considered each other their best friend. The friendship became romantic several years later.

Within several months of dating, they moved in together and enjoyed a committed relationship marked by emotional intimacy and stability. After five years, they decided to start a family and adopt a child. In an effort to prepare they both had complete physicals, including HIV tests. Although they both felt confident they would test negative, they felt they should get tested just to make absolutely sure.

Mike tested HIV positive. There was a period of acute shock, lasting for several weeks. In many ways, Claude appeared more devastated by Mike's diagnosis than Mike. He was anxious and frightened about Mike's overall prognosis and found it difficult to be apart from him. They called each other throughout their work days, checking on how each was feeling physically and emotionally. While Claude seemed to carry all the anxiety for the couple, Mike responded with depression. The more depressed Mike seemed, the more anxious Claude became. In the evenings, it was difficult for them to "just hang out." Mike felt smothered and constantly reminded of his HIV status. "I became my HIV" to Claude, he said. They came into therapy because they both felt they were drifting apart and did not understand why or how to find their way back to each other and how they were before the HIV diagnosis.

When conceptualizing a case such as this, noncognitive focused couple therapy provides a particularly useful set of constructs about the intrapsychic process between partners. It can also help us to with practice principles that are inherently systemic when looking at shifts in emotional intimacy between the partners; how interactional cycles promote behavioral patterns that foster fluctuating intimacy. The intrapsychic process for Mike and Claude included their own unique conflicts about this attachment and anticipated illness and the potential for psychological injury to the security of their attachment in the form of the HIV diagnosis. Based on this construct, assessment would focus on the underlying shifts in their emotional needs for intimacy and how Mike and Claude could turn their feelings into interactional positions by carrying out certain behaviors. These behaviors may belie preexisting conflicts about early attachments, and may be aimed at trying to repair or repeat their primary attachment patterns.

Emotionally focused assessment and de-escalation (steps 1-4) would go on to identify the problematic interactional cycle that maintains attachment insecurity and relationship distress, facilitating the partner's unacknowledged emotions and reframing their conflict so they can better understand and negotiate their behavioral patterns and attachment needs (Johnson, 1999).

Transcript excerpts and case analysis of the first stage of work with this couple follow:

MIKE: I'm feeling more and more like I can't really talk to him because everything I say, even if it's a small matter, he's obsessively worried. I don't want to worry him with anything so I don't tell him anything anymore.

THERAPIST: Would you say you feel like you have to protect Claude?

MIKE: Yeah. I feel like he's more freaked out by my diagnosis than I am.

THERAPIST: In the rare moments that you do feel worried or freaked out, what would you feel you need from him?

MIKE: I'd like to turn to him I guess. But it's not worth it. Then I have to take care of him. He's the one that's all freaked out. He should talk to his therapist or his friends, not me.

THERAPIST: Claude, what's your perspective on this pattern between you guys?

CLAUDE: I know he's right, but I'm just trying to show him my attentiveness . . . my concern, to support him so he doesn't feel alone with it.

THERAPIST: So Claude, your intention is to take care of Mike, to help him feel less alone, but Mike, when Claude pays special attention since the diagnosis, it feels like what?

MIKE: Like he's waiting for me to get sick and now I'm afraid if I ever do, he won't be able to handle it.

THERAPIST: So we have Claude trying to show his support in all good faith, but by the time it gets to you Mike, his attentiveness feels more like nervousness that makes you worry he may not be strong enough to provide strength for you if you should need it?

MIKE: Yeah. I hate saying that because I know his heart is in the right place, but I do worry that he's just too anxious now. God forbid something with my health really does happen. I fear he'd really break down.

THERAPIST: Given that this is how you feel, how does it make you behave toward Claude?

MIKE: Like I said. I don't tell him anything anymore and I keep things more to myself.

THERAPIST: Claude, when Mike behaves this way, how do you think you respond?

CLAUDE: I know how I respond. I get very hurt that he's shutting me out . . . and I try to get closer to him. I mean, are we a couple or aren't we?

This excerpt highlights the emotional and behavioral positioning and the therapist's effort to assess how emotions inform behavioral posturing for this couple. As Claude pursues intimacy with Mike, Mike backs away. This intensifies until they feel estranged and bewildered. There is also the attempt to de-escalate the conflict by helping each partner to better understand the difference between intent and affect. It is not Claude's intent to smother Mike with nervousness, but rather to show him moral support. It is not Mike's intent to hurt Claude, but rather a mechanism of self-protection. This highlights a common pattern of shifts in emotional intimacy that intensified after the HIV diagnosis. As each partner copes with a range of emotional reactions, it is not uncommon that as a unit, the couple may symmetrically move through stages in which they report feeling very close after the diagnosis and then more distant. In this particular scenario, the HIV diagnosis intensified a more unbalanced emotional pattern. Mike and Claude were at different end points on the continuum of emotional intimacy need in the face of Mike's diagnosis. Claude had always pursued a deeper emotional intimacy with Mike, and Mike had always been reluctant. Since the HIV diagnosis, Mike required more emotional distance ("feeling mercifully detached") and this intensified Claude's need for more intimacy and security ("I need to feel close to him, now more than ever"). Highlighting this to both partners diminishes the acute frustration and builds further empathy between them.

The therapist can move through this stage when the couple has a renewed empathic connection and an ability to understand their roles in their emotional and behavioral sequences. As their ability to understand each other and empathize with each other improves, the worker can guide the process to underlying emotions and underlying attachment issues both partners hold.

THERAPIST: Is there anything about the way this has played out that feels familiar from previous relationships or your families?

CLAUDE: That's just the way I deal with it. I've had to deal with illness my whole life. My mother, my sister. I'm not gonna break down. I just do better if I know everything, have all the information and can make decisions before a crisis comes. I'm not gonna break down. I'm just the worrying type. I deal with my worries by talking about them.

MIKE: Well I don't.

THERAPIST: So this is a significant difference between the two of you—how you cope with this sort of stress. Maybe before we figure out what might need to shift, and what might just need to be accepted or tolerated, can we hear from you Mike, what your needs are about this?

MIKE: I don't know. I guess I'm not used to this at all. My family never talked about anything and when we finally did, it was a disaster. It just makes me feel like I can't just be myself, that Claude looks at me and sees only my HIV. It feels terrible.

THERAPIST: So, both of you are operating as you always have, how you were taught in and by your families. Claude, you're feeling frightened and concerned for Mike . The way you deal with that is to pursue information, try to pay extra attention to Mike and to feel closer to him. Does that sound right?

CLAUDE: Yeah. It does.

THERAPIST: Mike, you're used to dealing with your emotions more on your own and you need a little more space and a little less emphasis on your HIV diagnosis and health? Does that feel accurate?

MIKE: Exactly. That's exactly how I feel.

THERAPIST: So in a way, the HIV brought out some of your different needs and styles about being close. Can we look at how to create a safe space between the two of you that allows for a balance of some emotional intimacy and some space when needed by either of you?

Although assessment and de-escalation will continue throughout in response to the couple's needs, the middle stages can begin with the creation of more adaptive interactional patterns. At this juncture, the therapist relying on EFCT enters a middle stage marked by the facilitation of changing maladaptive interactional behaviors and positioning. With further insight-oriented interventions, the respective partners are assisted in identifying disowned needs, promoting acceptance between both partners of these disowned emotional needs, and creating the empathic joining in the development of specifically different interactional behaviors that foster emotional engagement. A primary restructuring intervention in this phase is reframing in the

context of attachment needs, identifying and enacting more emotionally responsive behaviors (Johnson, 1999).

THERAPIST: Claude, what happens for you when Mike shuts down?

CLAUDE: I feel terrible. I feel like I don't know who he is when he's so distant. Sometimes I look at him and wonder whether he's really happy with me.

THERAPIST: You start to feel insecure about the future of your connection? Can we talk about what it is you need from Mike?

CLAUDE: I just need him to be more present, to be invested in me and in us. I feel like since the diagnosis, he's in his own world.

MIKE: You're insecure to begin with, and honestly I think no matter what I do you'll feel insecure. Any distance I need, you assume I'm mad . . . and you assume I'm mad at you. Sometimes I'm just quiet, I just don't feel like talking about this. It's something that makes me want to be alone.

THERAPIST: Maybe we can start to look at this a bit differently. What happens between the two of you is a dynamic that you both create. As Mike experiences painful feelings, he tends to withdraw a bit. As he withdraws, Claude you begin [to] feel anxious. Your anxiety makes you try to pull him back by proving your concern about his health since the diagnosis. But when you try to be closer with him in this way, it makes him very self-conscious about his diagnosis and worried about protecting you from further anxiety. The two of you have created a cycle in which neither is really feeling secure to get their emotional needs met.

This reflection provides Mike and Claude with a sense of a shared responsibility for this problematic dynamic. It also reframes the nature of this conflict away from their behavioral positions and toward their underlying emotions and needs within this attachment. The final stage includes the consolidation and integration of new interactional positioning of each partner that encourages more mutually satisfying attachment experiences in a more stable manner as opposed to wide swings in emotional intimacy.

THERAPIST: Now, feeling a clearer understanding of what each of you has been feeling, how might things change to meet both of your needs?

CLAUDE: If he can reassure me that he will take good care of himself and be honest with me when he's not feeling well, I can try and back up.

MIKE: Ok. I can deal with that. But if I'm honest, then you have to be less focused on this. Can't you ask me how my day was, without always asking me how I feel?

CLAUDE: I'll try. But, can you try not to be so distant. Let me know what you're thinking, how you're feeling?
MIKE: I can try. It'll depend on how you react.

With a deeper understanding and appreciation of each other's needs, Mike and Claude developed a new set of expectations about how to meet their different needs for emotional intimacy. These excerpts highlight how to intervene to de-escalate a destructive interactional pattern about different emotional needs, build empathy between partners, and develop more adaptive behavioral patterns around shifting emotional needs in response to an HIV diagnosis.

SUMMARY

As Bowlby (1969) and Bowen's (1978) theories would assert, in every couple there is the constant unconscious tension between establishing close attachment ties and the innate need to individuate. How can each individual balance the conflict of merging versus individuation when his or her relationship is impacted by HIV? Couples facing the threat of chronic or acute illness may experience emotional reactions on a continuum with each other that spans from enmeshment to emotional disengagement from each other.

Borrowing from medical family therapy, the experience of diagnosis is a nodal event for the dyad that will shift both functional and emotional positioning in relation to each partner. The diagnosis of HIV may incur a centrifugal response, pulling the couple away from each other. The emotional reactions to HIV diagnosis may also have a centripetal force pushing the couple toward each other. In some instances, the couple will manifest different drives at different times to be drawn together in a renewed and more meaningful commitment and also experience periods of ambivalence and impulses away from each other in the face of the diagnosis. For some, this pushing and pulling apart becomes a dynamic in which one or both partners experience anxiety in response to increased levels of emotional intimacy and attachment, and the couple creates an emotional experience to diffuse the intimacy and allow for distance.

The language of serodiscordance, being referred to as HIV positive and HIV negative, induces and exacerbates feelings of disengagement between partners. The serodiscordance can sometimes be used as a mask representing or deflecting underlying feelings of emotional disengagement. The reverse is also to be pursued—that conflict around day-to-day differences, housekeeping, can be used by the couple to mask underlying feelings of estrangement evoked by the serodiscordance.

Chapter 8

Impact of Uncertainty

"Since the diagnosis, we never feel sure about our future. It's like every day, every doctor's appointment can change everything."

OVERVIEW

Adapting to the uncertainty of any physical illness has long been a documented primary task for patients and their family members (Moos and Tsu, 1977). Many couples living with an acute illness live with a high sense of vigilance, that each moment or day may bring a new symptom signaling an impending loss.

Although the length of time between an HIV diagnosis and the first symptoms of an opportunistic infection has now extended, the emotional experience of living with uncertainty continues to be a common and profound challenge for individuals and couples (CDC, 2001; Mancilla and Troshinsky, 2003). The experience of uncertainty about disease progression is drastically different for different communities, as people of color and women continue to have a much shorter period between testing HIV positive and becoming symptomatic because they have fewer opportunities for access to an expansive range of social and medical supports.

Medical family systems theory identifies the common experience of anxiety a family lives with after a diagnosis, and even during periods of remission. Often, nervous anticipation of a return to illness haunts the couple even as the HIV-positive partner seems to be asymptomatic. The trauma of diagnosis leaves many families acutely aware and anxious of a potential reoccurrence of illness that will rob their loved ones of their health and emotional security. Living with the uncertainty of an illness presenting itself on any given day and not knowing whether the illness can be treated effectively is a common emotional challenge for any family living with the reality of chronic or acute medical illness. However, some unique dimensions of uncertainty exist for a couple of mixed HIV status.

QUANTITATIVE FINDINGS

The majority of couples (74 percent, n = 61) living with one partner diagnosed with HIV report that uncertainty is a primary challenge intrapsychically and within the relationship.

Uncertainty was referred to around three distinct phenomena. Uncertainty regarding how the virus might progress was the most commonly defined issue. Respondents provided examples of this in their responses to open-ended questions, such as: "We never know from day to day, how his viral load may change, get worse or better. We're just forever in limbo about how the disease will or won't progress."

Responses that reflected uncertainty included questions about how long they or their partner would be HIV asymptomatic, how treatable an infection might be, and if and how one might tolerate side effects from their combination therapies. These issues are not unique to couples living with medical illness, but given the swiftly changing nature of our understanding of HIV infection, progression, and treatment, uncertainty is an unremitting companion for couples of mixed HIV status.

The second area of uncertainty was about how long the negative partner will continue to test negative and how they might cope if "God forbid, she gets it too," as one boyfriend stated. A wife characterized this area of uncertainty in the following way: "We know I have it. That's about the only known thing we know for sure. Every day, we wonder what if he gets it too. It's an unspoken tension."

This comment is a segue into the third area of uncertainty, which can be described as an uncertainty about whether their negative partners will be able to see them through the end of their illness. For example, one woman noted, "He's okay now that I'm not sick, but if I get really sick, I don't know if he can take it and will be able to stay and take care of me."

These three strands of uncertainty were expressed by both HIV-positive and HIV-negative respondents. As with any chronic illness, a specter of the unknown about disease progression and caretaking anxieties exists. In addition to these uncertainties, there is the unique unknown of HIV transmission and how the couple would deal with the potential reality of both testing HIV positive or both becoming ill.

Coping with the uncertainty provoked by the HIV diagnosis was shared by gay and straight couples alike. The only notable distinction is that those partners in a straight relationship appeared to feel somewhat more strongly that uncertainty was a primary concern in their relationship than their counterparts in gay-identified relationships, as seen in Table 8.1.

Uncertainty, in all its forms, was experienced more often as a primary concern for females than for males. Eighty-five percent of women in serodiscordant relationships reported that uncertainty was a primary concern, whereas only 64 percent of men strongly agreed that uncertainty was a primary concern. In fact, 11 percent of men reported that uncertainty due to HIV in their relationships presented no concern for themselves and their partners. This highlights that women tend to experience, or at least choose to articulate, the anxiety around all the possible uncertainties an HIV diagnosis may portend. This concurs with Van der Straten et al. (1998) and Kennedy et al.'s (1995) findings that women in serodiscordant couples report higher levels of emotional distress, regardless of who is living with the HIV diagnosis, than do their male partners (see Table 8.2).

Women, whether they were the partner who had tested HIV positive or the partner who had tested negative, tended to feel more distress from the uncertainty that the diagnosis brought into the relation-

TABLE 8.1. Sexual orientation: Uncertainty is of primary concern.

	Strongly agree	Agree	Disagree	Strongly disagree	Total
Heterosexual	36 (75%)	11 (23%)	1 (2%)	0	48
Homosexual	25 (62.5%)	8 (20%)	7 (17.5%)	0	40
Total	61	19	8	0	88

ship. Men, particularly those who were HIV-negative, seemed to experience slightly less distress than their female HIV-negative counterparts. Admittedly, this is based on a very small sample, but perhaps future research can further investigate the reliability of the slight pattern demonstrated in Table 8.3.

Essentially, uncertainty provoked by the HIV diagnosis in a relationship appeared to be experienced equally across the three ethnicities represented in this study. Sixty-five percent of African Americans, 75 percent of Hispanics, and 67 percent of white respondents

TABLE 8.2. Gender in heterosexual relationships: Uncertainty is of primary concern.

	Strongly agree	Agree	Disagree	Strongly disagree	Total
Female	17 (85%)	3 (15%)	0	0	20
Male	44 (65%)	16 (23%)	8 (12%)	0	68
Total	61	19	8	0	88

TABLE 8.3. HIV-positive partners in heterosexual relationships: Uncertainty is of primary concern.

	Strongly agree	Agree	Disagree	Strongly disagree	Total
HIV-positive women	8 (80%)	2 (20%)	0	0	10
HIV-positive men	6 (60%)	3 (30%)	1 (10%)	0	10
HIV-negative women	9 (90%)	1 (10%)	0	0	10
HIV-negative men	4 (40%)	3 (30%)	3 (30%)	0	10
Total	27	9	4	0	40

strongly agreed that uncertainty had become a primary concern in their relationships due to the HIV diagnosis. African-American couples seemed to experience the least upset regarding uncertainty, and, in fact, 22 percent reported that they did not experience uncertainty as a primary concern as seen in Table 8.4.

Not surprising, those partners who were living with the positive HIV diagnosis reported that uncertainty was more a primary concern in the relationship (82 percent) than their partners who remained HIV negative (57 percent) (Table 8.5). The three different scenarios of uncertainty that emerged from the narrative responses included uncertainty about the course of the illness, uncertainty about whether the HIV-negative partner would seroconvert, and uncertainty about whether the HIV-negative partner would be able to care for his or her part-

TABLE 8.4. Ethnicity: Uncertainty is of primary concern.

	Strongly agree	Agree	Disagree	Strongly disagree	Total
African American	15 (65%)	3 (13%)	5 (22%)	0	23
Hispanic	21 (75%)	5 (18%)	2 (7%)	0	28
White	25 (67%)	11 (30%)	1 (3%)	0	37
Total	61	19	8	0	88

TABLE 8.5. Serostatus: Uncertainty is of primary concern.

	Strongly agree	Agree	Disagree	Strongly disagree	Total
HIV positive	36 (82%)	5 (11%)	3 (7%)	0	44
HIV negative	25 (57%)	14 (32%)	5 (11%)	0	44
Total	61	19	8	0	88

ner should they become ill. Given the third category of uncertainty, it is clear why those testing positive experienced higher levels of uncertainty than their partners.

As with every issue identified in this study, the length of a couple's relationship has been an important predictor (Table 8.6). The longer a couple has been together, the better the couple seems to cope with each challenge raised by HIV in the relationship. As in this case, the longer the couples have been together, the less uncertainty was reported as a primary concern. Eighty-four percent of those couples who have been together less than five years reported uncertainty as a primary concern in their relationship. Compare this to the 58 percent of couples who have been together for more than five years who reported the same. Although this is not always the case, as many couples stay together longer, they may have developed more stable and resilient coping patterns with numerous challenges prior to the HIV diagnosis. In newer relationships, however, there may be a general aura of uncertainty about the viability of their future together, and this may be exacerbated by the HIV diagnosis more readily than in a longer-term relationship.

As the length of a relationship has proved to be a predictor, so too has the timing of when the couple learned of the diagnosis (Table 8.7). For those couples who knew of their serodiscordance from the start of their courtship, uncertainty played a significantly less disruptive role than those who learned of the diagnosis later in an established relationship. Thirty-four percent of those who knew of the diagnosis coming into the relationship identified uncertainty as a primary concern in the relationship, whereas 71 percent of those couples

TABLE 8.6. Length of relationship: Uncertainty is of primary concern.

	Strongly agree	Agree	Disagree	Strongly disagree	Total
Less than 5 years	32 (84%)	4 (11%)	2 (5%)	0	38
More than 5 years	29 (58%)	15 (30%)	6 (12%)	0	50
Total	61	19	8	0	88

who learned of the diagnosis after the relationship was established reported uncertainty as a primary concern.

Eighty-one percent of couples who experienced an HIV-related illness strongly agreed that uncertainty was a primary area of concern in the relationship, versus 55 percent of couples in relationships that have not experienced HIV-related illness (Table 8.8). Research in medical family therapy indicates that for those families that have experienced a medical crisis, they often remain at the ready, suffering from an anticipatory anxiety about the unknown of when a relapse might occur and how severe it may be. Clearly, the reality of going through a medical crisis left couples more unsettled and perhaps more attuned to their feelings about living with the uncertainty HIV may bring.

TABLE 8.7. When couple learned of HIV diagnosis: Uncertainty is of primary concern.

	Strongly agree	Agree	Disagree	Strongly disagree	Total
Diagnosed before relationship	11 (34%)	13 (41%)	8 (25%)	0	32
Diagnosed in relationship	40 (71%)	16 (29%)	0	0	56
Total	51	29	8	0	88

TABLE 8.8. HIV-related illness: Uncertainty is of primary concern.

	Strongly agree	Agree	Disagree	Strongly disagree	Total
Have had HIV illness	39 (81%)	9 (19%)	0	0	48
Have not had HIV illness	22 (55%)	10 (25%)	8 (20%)	0	40
Total	61	19	8	0	88

QUALITATIVE FINDINGS

Narrative Responses

Uncertainty About Course of Illness

"We never know whether the next time he gets sick will be more serious."

"I know on some level, when we talk about planning our future, even summer plans, we both wonder, what if I get sick?"

"Just because he's responding well to the treatment now, doesn't mean it'll continue to work. We have a lot of friends who had to be taken off the triple combination meds."

"Yeah, the meds are working now, but we know I can fall like many before me at any time, so we don't ever feel secure that I'll continue to be healthy."

"When my boyfriend gets any type of a cold, even a sore throat or just feels under the weather, we're both terrified that this is the beginning of the end. It's hard to know when we're overreacting and when we'll get caught with a medical crisis."

"I'd like to think I can tolerate these side effects, but I'm not sure I'll be able. Without them [the medicines], I just don't know how I'll do."

"My husband is so nervous about my health, that we don't really do anything anymore because he's afraid if I tax myself, I'll get sick. It makes us feel like we're not really able to live life because we're so uncertain about my health."

"We've been so lucky he's still asymptomatic. I know at some point he won't be. We just don't know when."

"I've had a few infections already, so now we feel like the next one can come at any time and it makes us feel like we're living with something hanging over us all the time."

Uncertainty About Ability of HIV-Negative Partner to Care for HIV-Positive Partner

"We don't talk to each other about it, but I know we both worry what would happen if I got really sick . . . would he be able to take care of me? . . ."

"I know my husband loves me deeply, but I also worry he won't be able to see me getting sick or being sick. I just feel insecure about it."

"I will always be with my partner no matter what, but I think he feels uncertain about whether I'll be able to take care of him if he gets sick, not emotionally, but all the other ways—negotiating [with] doctors and everything."

"I think he tries to take care of everything to show me he can be depended on if I'm sick. I think we both feel unsteady about what would happen if I can't take care of stuff the way I always have."

Uncertainty About Conversion of HIV-Negative Partner

"The thing we've been feeling worried about is what if we both end up positive. Then everything's up for grabs. Anything can happen to both of us."

"We worry that even if we're practicing safer sex, what if I still get the AIDS virus from him. I feel like there's always some unlucky bastard, y'know the condom breaks or something. I just feel we can never be sure that I'll stay negative."

"What if I get it from him? He doesn't like to always use a condom. . . . I don't know what we'd do if I get it also."

"We've tried to be careful, but I think we both feel like it's possible that I could've gotten it and could get it."

Case Studies

Case I: Louisa and Frank

Louisa is a thirty-seven-year-old West Indian and African-American woman with a long history of alcohol, cocaine, and IV heroin use. She comes from a working-class family, and was raised by her mother and grandmother. Her father left her mother when the children were young, and Louisa was told by the adults in her family that he left because "he wasn't a family man." From the ages of nine through thirteen, Louisa was sexually molested by her brother and a male cousin. When she spoke up about this at age thirteen, her mother told her not to tell anyone.

By age seventeen, Louisa drank regularly and had begun experimenting with cocaine. She describes her adolescence and young adulthood as chaotic and depressed. She had many relationships with both men and women, and after a ten-year abusive relationship with her first husband, she left him at age thirty-three. After what seemed like an unusually long flu she couldn't recover from, she was treated and tested for HIV. She tested positive two and one-half years ago. She has been clean and sober for two years and reports that now that she is sober, she would like to learn how to cope with her

HIV within the context of her relationship with Frank, her partner of three years. Her chief complaint is that she feels they are stuck in a limbo of uncertainty. She reports that they never plan for the future and are both unable to live in the moment for fear that she will become acutely ill at any time.

Frank is a forty-seven-year-old West Indian man who was raised in Jamaica and came with his father to the United States when he was ten years old. His immigration was most difficult, leaving his loving mother behind and living with his hardened father who made excessive demands on him. Frank has always relied on alcohol and marijuana to help him relax and "feel better." He had a history as a loner until he was forced to enter Narcotics Anonymous (NA) and Alcoholics Anonymous (AA) as a condition for keeping his job at a community hospital. Frank thrived in recovery. He enjoyed his sobriety, his socialization, and his relationship with Louisa as she became sober as well. Frank says he is deeply in love with Louisa and worries all the time that she will become ill and he is unable to think about anything else but the uncertainty of her health.

This couple presented as depressed and unable to mobilize themselves, both individually and as a couple. They wanted help to "break out" of their depression about the diagnosis. In assessment, both partners demonstrated great motivation to improve the quality of their life together, seemed to share a tender and loving connection, but were emotionally incapacitated by the diagnosis. Time stopped, especially for Frank, the day Louisa tested positive. All the motivation they shared to "treasure their time together even more" could not be realized.

Frank was initially angry and disbelieving of the diagnosis, and subsequently has been despairing at times. He seemed to be in a perpetual state of anticipatory grief. This is a state marked by preoccupation and mourning about an impending loss. Louisa had some ability to accept her diagnosis and try to move on, but when Frank was not able to share her optimism, she despaired.

They both became despairing and were not able to reintegrate emotionally or functionally after her diagnosis. The usual routines they had were different—the way they spent time together, the things they talked about—all changed after the diagnosis. There was a distinct sense of before and after since the diagnosis, and both felt confusion, isolation, and sadness. Louisa was referred by her clinical case manager to meet with a couple counselor because she and Frank seemed to be struggling so much since the diagnosis. This case required a truly integrated framework that consisted of multiple approaches and borrowed interventions that could shore up their worry and pain. Initially, medical family therapy was the most responsive approach. A primary theoretical premise of medical family therapy is that when any individual is diagnosed with an illness, it can most fully be assessed and intervened with by working with the entire family. The family is the most potent strength and stressor in a medical crisis, and to truly aid the individual with the new diagnosis, the family must be helped to become more of a strength and less of a stressor. McDaniel et al. (1995) identified the four primary aims of medical family therapy as: (1) advocating patient and family to be fully educated about their health status, (2) facilitating open communication between family members about the illness, (3) helping family to adjust to new functional and emotional roles, and (4) helping patient and family to develop effective coping and adaptation to the diagnosis and illness. One could not move to enjoin them empathetically until much of this work had been effectively completed. The components of this approach that were essential to building a foundation for future couple treatment on a deeper level included psychoeducation and development of mutual aid support for each partner.

As Frank and Louisa spoke about the diagnosis, it was evident that neither had a full understanding of the diagnosis, prognosis, and treatment options. In fact, a small part of their depression and anxiety lifted as we looked at the difference between their respective fantasies of living with HIV and the present reality of living with HIV. The current medical updates provided significantly more optimistic views of their future than either had believed. When they were told of the diagnosis, like many people, they experienced a form of shock. They both said they were flooded with the pictures and images from newspapers and television of those dying of AIDS in Africa. Although rationally they both knew Louisa may not be in imminent danger such as that, they could not shake the terror of those images.

Louisa's physician and an HIV counselor provided them with information and education, but they realize now, almost two years later, that they "didn't hear a word they said." This is surely not uncommon, and has to be part of counseling anyone who has been diagnosed with any potentially serious illness. The case manager assumed Louisa had been able to take in this information and never returned to it, but rather moved onto more mundane business regarding her care.

The need for additional support to this couple was self-evident. Social support networks needed to be identified and facilitated. This brought up the dilemma of disclosure (to be discussed in detail in Chapter 9), but with encouragement they were able to tell key family members and friends and found a reconnection with their church as well. Further, they each became part of a group for support in different agencies. For Frank, this was essential and critical to his return to the relationship. He began to talk about what he was going through at NA and AA and at his new support group, and he could not believe how generously and compassionately he was received and supported.

With these social supports in place and working effectively, the couple's overall coping and adaptation improved. They reported how helpful their fellowship and support was around coping with the diagnosis. The next area of focus was to open up their communication with each other about Louisa's illness.

THERAPIST: In some ways, you've both been able to talk to others more easily than to each other. Can we look at what you need to be able to talk honestly with each other about the diagnosis?

LOUISA: I don't know.

FRANK: I couldn't say.

THERAPIST: What makes it difficult for you to talk to each other about this?

LOUISA: I don't want to upset him.

THERAPIST: Frank, Louisa says she doesn't want to talk to you because she doesn't want to upset you. What do you think of that?

FRANK: I think that's silly. It's me that should be protecting her. I don't want her to have to hear my worries because it will bring her more stress. I feel guilty to give her any stress when her health is fragile to begin with.

THERAPIST: What if she would like to be able to talk to you about her feelings about her diagnosis and what she worries about? What if by talking to you, she unburdened herself and felt less stressed? Can she lean on you that way?

LOUISA: He's got enough on his mind. I'll talk to other people. I don't want to worry him.

THERAPIST: [Knowing of Louisa's history as a parentified child and someone forced to hold her secret, this pattern seemed consistent.] Louisa, how would it feel if you didn't have to keep your feelings secret from Frank?

FRANK: I don't want her to keep anything secret from me. I want to ease her burden anyway I can.

LOUISA: [Weeping] I'm so sorry. I'm so sorry I'm a burden now.

This poignant exchange activated both partners emotionally and allowed their internal processes to be seen and experienced by each other. In some ways this dialogue reflects the heart of medical family therapy—opening communication about illness between patient and family—but it also opened an empathic connection, which is at the heart of emotionally focused couple therapy. The feeling in the room changed dramatically once Louisa expressed how she felt and Frank showed her he understood and cared. This defining moment in treatment ushered in more emotionally focused work about how they both had experienced the diagnosis and how they could be closer through all this uncertainty. With their emotional needs identified, both for more intimacy through this time of uncertainty, we were able to pursue a greater understanding of how their underlying attachment issues and conflicts (fear of betrayal for Louisa) were exacerbated by the uncertainty surrounding her health. Bowlby's (1969) research led to the conclusion that in sickness and calamity adults experience primary attachment behaviors. This was demonstrated in the next portion of the transcript from Louisa and Frank.

FRANK: I just lost all hope after the diagnosis. I thought I was going to lose her.

LOUISA: He's just never been able to get over it. I think he still lives in that day each day. He doesn't see that I'm okay. At least for now. He's waiting for me to get sick, every day.

THERAPIST: Frank, what do you think? How have you been coping with not knowing about Louisa's future?

FRANK: [Long pause and heavy sighs.] I'm really scared. I just don't think we should forget just because she's feeling better. I feel we should prepare ourselves. In my family, we never did. I lost my grandma. She died after a long illness when I was five and my family was ruined. [Long silence.] I don't know. I never thought about it in this way, but in a way I lost my mother when my father took me here and it was a surprise. I just always felt like if we had known, we could've been better prepared.

THERAPIST: These losses seem connected to your wish to stay vigilant now. What do you think you learned about yourself through these losses?

FRANK: What did I learn? I learned to keep it to myself and that it's better to prepare somehow for the unknown otherwise you give up. I'm either all guns forward or I give up.

LOUISA: Did you hear yourself just now? Did you hear that that's exactly how you're behaving? Like you gave up the day I got diagnosed.

One way of understanding this complex dynamic is that Frank's formative experiences with attachment and loss were a blueprint for his adult relationships. This is a man who experienced almost textbook emotional responses to loss; the three phases of protest, despair, and finally disengagement were described with the passing of his grandmother and then again in leaving his mother at a young age. Another way of understanding his withdrawing was somewhat more dynamic in nature. After Louisa's diagnosis, she reported that she felt Frank could not cope with her feelings of sadness and worry, and she protected him by emotionally withdrawing. For Louisa, this was consistent with her primary relationship with her mother, one that was characterized by a defining sense that her mother could not take care of her emotionally, and so she withdrew in response. This was a pattern in the type of partner she sought out: one that was unable to share her emotional pain and someone who would tolerate her withdrawal.

Given Frank and Louisa's histories, the circular positioning was set in place: as she withdrew, his sense of loss intensified and he became even more despairing. As uncertainty about her health presented itself, Louisa felt she could not burden Frank, and he felt he could not tolerate anticipating her illness. Each insight that emerged in session was only a hypothesis, and as is often the case the couple looked for one right answer. The notion of a multifaceted view to each conflict was a way of removing the familiar patterns of mutual accusation.

Fostering such insights regarding Frank's attachment needs and his attachment issues enabled the couple to move ahead with greater clarity about Frank's behavior in response to the uncertainty provoked by Louisa's HIV diagnosis. Understanding some of these complexities at play for Frank, Louisa was enabled to open up toward him in kind.

THERAPIST: Louisa you seem to really feel for Frank. Can you help him understand what's happened for you since the diagnosis? How you've coped with the uncertainties surrounding your health?

LOUISA: I guess I'm more mixed than him. I feel shocked and sometimes even hopeless, but then I also feel like I don't want to give up. I mean, I may have to someday, it may even be soon, but all this time, so far, we're kind of wasting. I want to do stuff together. I want to enjoy what time I have. Even if I get sick soon, I can't really believe it. . . . feel okay, and I don't want to look back and regret this time that I did have my health, that we could have enjoyed our time together, but he's so full of sadness and anger. [Frank sits and avoids looking at Louisa with his head down.]

THERAPIST: Frank, are you able to let Louisa know that you heard what she goes through? [He only nods.]

LOUISA: *[Frustrated]* This is why I don't talk to him. He doesn't want to hear. He says he does, but if I really tell him, he doesn't.

THERAPIST: And that makes you feel, what?

LOUISA: Like a fool for trying. I don't think he can hear it and I should have trusted my intuition.

After a brief discussion, Louisa sees that her "intuition" has also been formed by her previous experiences with risking her vulnerability, seeking someone to be emotionally supportive, and then being disappointed in her relationship with her mother. Frank is enlisted as an active listener as she retells what she has learned about attachments, depending on others and protecting others. He is helped to understand how his behaviors are cues to her to protect him and that she may feel unable to depend on him for emotional support. This reflects EFCT's focus on how partners create their ongoing experiences with each other and how these rigid patterns repeat until a deeper understanding of underlying emotions can provide an emotional breakthrough for the couple that will result in shifted interactional dynamics.

That's all that Louisa needed to hear. With a combination of medical family therapy and EFCT, a foundation of honest communication and renewed emotional intimacy with each other was being built. Luckily, this couple was highly motivated and capable of risking themselves with each other. Establishing and consolidating more adaptive behaviors between each other had yet to be completed.

THERAPIST: So you've both drawn away in different ways and for sort of similar reasons, to protect each other and yourselves. Maybe we can start to look at what each of you needs to feel bold enough to risk more intimacy.

LOUISA: I just have to know that I'm not burdening him, and that he can let some good feelings in some time. If he's always miserable, it makes me frustrated.

THERAPIST: Frank, what would you need from her to give her this?

FRANK: She's gotta let me be upset sometimes. She's gotta give me a chance to be strong for her.

They identified how these needs could be translated into behaviors that both recognized as different, more open, and more trusting. They continued to struggle, particularly Frank with depression. Overall, they reported significant improvement in their relationship, and left after eight sessions saying they felt more confident they could "get through this together."

Case II: Kevin and Anthony

To illustrate another perspective on uncertainty, we will revisit the case of Kevin and Anthony that was discussed in Chapter 6 regarding fear of HIV transmission. This couple had weathered several potential breakups due to Kevin's infidelity and settled into a stable and mutually satisfying relationship over the past four years. This changed again when Kevin's HIV test came back positive. With this, they both experienced acute anxiety and intense and unremitting fighting. There was intense anger on Anthony's part who was furious about Kevin "bringing this virus into their home." They could not decide whether they were able to remain together given this injury, and given the uncertainty about the security of their relationship that preexisted the diagnosis. They sought couple counseling, reporting that their relationship was "in serious trouble," and they thought they'd like to try and save it if they could. This was a couple with a preexisting pattern of chaos and crisis.

Kevin's diagnosis was the "hazardous event" crisis intervention theory describes as the occurrence that destabilizes an individual or a family. This event created enough stress in this dyad that it threatened the couple's stability. As they described the day of diagnosis and the weeks that followed, they described thoughts, feelings, and behaviors that could only be defined as active crisis. They moved through a vulnerable state marked by an inability to cope. Their efforts to cope included an agreement to avoid acknowledging the diagnosis, an effort to talk frankly about the diagnosis, and every combination of denial and confrontation in between. They presented in a full state of crisis in their relationship and as individuals.

The central goal of crisis theory is to facilitate more effective coping mechanisms to better adapt to the real and perceived loss of a particular event. The initial interventions are aimed relief of emotional turmoil, restoration of precrisis functioning (unsettled at best in this scenario), fuller understanding of how events contributed to crisis state, identification of resources, and recognition between present stress and previous life losses. These practice principles are delivered through sustainment, clarification ventilation, and provision of concrete services in an effort to equip, usually our individual, with more adaptive coping techniques. In this case, we have two individuals in crisis and a relationship in crisis.

According to Parad (1965), three patterns of adaptive crisis resolution exist: (1) correct/accurate cognitive perception, (2) management of affect (acceptance/release of feelings, such as sadness, anger, and guilt), and (3) ability to seek and accept help. Can this be transferred from crisis intervention with an individual to crisis intervention with a dyad? Always relying on the three principles outlined by Ripple (1964), predictors of the client's motivation, capacity, and opportunity for benefitting from a helping relationship, assessment proceeded.

Initial stages could consist of nothing more than engagement with primary emphasis on ventilation (keeping it as constructive and conflict-free wherever possible) and sustainment. Kevin and Anthony were helped to tell their stories in ways that were different from their fighting patterns at home, which were typically in the classic accuse-accuse communication format. As their communication patterns included less accusations and more active listening, it was evident they were both deeply motivated to stay together as a couple, to "deal with the HIV," and to make every effort in couple counseling. They were both capable in terms of insight, but their high emotional reactivity would be an ongoing challenge.

The intense level of uncertainty and bitterness that had been swirling around this couple exploded when Kevin received his HIV diagnosis. Uncertainly existed on many levels, but the most pressing was whether they would remain a couple at all. Basic tools for coping needed to be provided to equip Kevin and Anthony to sit in the same room and not wish to destroy each other or feel destroyed in return.

Noting this as a potential obstacle to progress, early work focused simultaneously on de-escalation of maladaptive communication patterns and the implementation of coping tools. This included communication skills, such as active listening, paraphrasing, taking the "I stand," and development of empathic responses between partners. It also included cognitive interventions that aimed to provide them each with a clearer sense of how their thought patterns, sometimes based on mind reading, generalizing, and dichotomous thinking, resulted in nonproductive fights. Stress management was also introduced in session and as homework with such tools as deep breathing, muscle relaxation, and restructuring imagery so they can cope better with their intense feelings. (Stress management techniques such as these have been found to significantly enhance the coping skills of those coping with the uncertainty surrounding HIV/AIDS, and their family members.)

After three sessions, Kevin and Anthony began to move out of their active crisis state. They moved toward reintegration, a phase marked by the beginning of acceptance of the changed situation and the development of more effective coping mechanisms. Individually, both had external resources for social support. In addition to couple counseling, Kevin was lucky enough to find a support group that had just started for newly diagnosed individuals. Anthony found support in his religious and spiritual circle of friends. In addition, both had told several friends and select family members and found that they felt relieved and supported by loved ones.

In session, they had agreed not to sever the relationship for at least four sessions. This also made both partners feel somewhat relieved. The many tools they were given for communication and stress management during this period of uncertainty proved to be relatively effective in stemming injurious fights.

As their rigid and destructive patterns of communication and behavior became more flexible and more constructive, it was critical to shore up their emotional engagement with each other. Although they experienced uncertainty about their relationship and about how HIV would affect their relationship, focus remained on de-escalating their crisis states, shoring up their internal and external resources, facilitating more adaptive coping mechanisms, and building more adaptive communication with each other. There were deep issues of mistrust and betrayal due to the HIV diagnosis and preexisting infidelities between Kevin and Anthony that were a primary obstacle in sustaining intimacy. These issues were addressed in later treatment.

SUMMARY

Coping with uncertainty for couples of mixed HIV status includes three primary areas of uncertainty. The first is coping with the unknown surrounding how the disease might progress, how long an HIV-negative partner will remain HIV negative, and how the couple will cope with acute or end-stage illness. There were also uncertainties voiced about how long a partner might be able to tolerate side effects of a medication regime and how one might manage if not able to tolerate such a regime.

Living with these different dimensions of uncertainty surrounding the presence of HIV in their relationship, couples experienced high levels of anxiety and stress internally and dyadically. It often manifested in an increase in fighting between partners about "day-to-day" issues since the diagnosis. In session, when couples were assisted to speak about the uncertainties and the feelings it engendered, they were more able to discuss it with each other than either partner imagined. Focusing initially on communication skills and then empathic joining, couples often improved their sense of emotional engagement and alliance. When partners were motivated and capable, they were able to shift patterns toward sharing their emotional experience of worry as opposed to withdrawing from each other or trying to protect their partners (which ultimately resulted in more emotional distance). The practitioner should anticipate that uncertainty will accompany a couple of mixed HIV status and should elicit how they have coped with so many important unknowns, individually and as a couple, and facilitate their joint coping patterns wherever possible.

Chapter 9

Disclosure Issues

"The worst part of this all, is that he won't tell anyone. I have no one to talk to because he's terrified of anybody finding out."

OVERVIEW

Disclosure to friends and family is associated with increased social support, and this support in turn has been proven to provide better quality of life and even quantity of life (Josephson, 1997). Overall, the stress of keeping the secret of HIV appears to be isolating, depressing, and more deleterious to the physical and emotional well-being of the individual, couple, and family (Hays et al., 1993). This is a particularly important issue to be cognizant of when assessing a couple of mixed HIV status (Josephson, 1997; Poindexter, 2004).

Disclosure issues include conflict about whether to disclose one's HIV status at all, when, and to whom. Other issues around disclosing HIV status to families of origin or shared friends may be conflictual for couples, such as the transmission source (gay or bisexual activity or drug injection use being among the most difficult) (Marks et al., 1992). Because HIV status affects both partners, one has to anticipate that the couple may have different needs about disclosing the positive HIV status in themself or their partner.

Given the unprecedented stigma that has surrounded HIV/AIDS in this and other countries, many individuals continue to feel trapped into silence about revealing their or their partner's positive HIV status. In the United States, HIV is still primarily contracted through homosexual contact and injection drug use, with heterosexual contact still the lesser source of these three transmission routes. The historical and current hostility and even violence against those with HIV/

AIDS have created an immense challenge to the individual and couple affected by HIV who struggle with who and when to disclose.

Regardless of sexual orientation or ethnic background, a balance between a shared marital identity and autonomous identity for each partner is tested once a partner's HIV status is disclosed to family, friends, or co-workers, as couples are often viewed as a couple with HIV. This can exacerbate any preexisting issues, developmental or characterological, about their internal and external boundaries, how they perceive themselves, and how they wish to be perceived by others regarding HIV.

For gay men, there can be a deep conflict about disclosing HIV status as it often entails a "double coming out" to family as HIV infected and as a gay man. For some the religious and cultural positions against homosexuality obstruct disclosing their HIV status, as this may result in loss of family of origin and perceived injury to their family of origin. With injection use, disclosing HIV status may include a double coming out if the drug use has been kept secret. This chapter identifies how couples experience this challenge and discusses which couples experience the most conflict around disclosing their mixed HIV status.

Earlier in the history of HIV/AIDS in the United States, disclosure appeared to be a more predominant issue for gay male couples than it is in the current era. In fact, Walker (1991) described why the "gay man" might keep his diagnosis secret: "[D]iagnosis with AIDS often triggers an eruption of self-doubt, reviving repressive, homophobic voices that the gay man has tried to subdue. . . . The patient who blames himself does not want to face his family or even the feared reproaches of disgust of a lover" (p. 31). This speaks to the "double coming out" or two tiers of stigma gay men with HIV/AIDS experience (Cadwell, 1991). However, this may be more reflective of the initial phases of the HIV epidemic as this and other current studies demonstrated that disclosure issues created more distress in heterosexual couples than it did in gay couples (Josephson, 1997).

QUANTITATIVE FINDINGS

Nearly 53 percent of heterosexual couples strongly agreed that disclosure was a primary concern in their relationship while only 17 percent of gay couples identified this as a primary issue in their relationship. In fact, 40 percent of gay couples disagreed that disclosure was problematic as seen in Table 9.1.

When exploring how disclosure was experienced differently according to gender, males and females voiced essentially the same levels of distress, with a third of both genders strongly agreeing that disclosure of HIV status was a primary concern (Table 9.2). However, as evidenced later in this chapter in narrative responses, it seemed that more women were frustrated by lack of disclosure in their male partners than vice versa.

Within heterosexual relationships, responses indicated that men and women, regardless of serostatus, struggled equally with disclosure issues. Disclosure of HIV status appeared to be the least stressful in those relationships in which the female was HIV negative as seen in Table 9.3. This finding concurs with Williams-Saporito (1998) and Mayer and Wells (1997) who found that the female in heterosexual

TABLE 9.1. Sexual orientation: Disclosure of HIV status is of primary concern.

	Strongly agree	Agree	Disagree	Strongly disagree	Total
Heterosexual	21 (52.5%)	15 (37.5%)	4 (10%)	0	40
Homosexual	8 (17%)	16 (33%)	19 (40%)	5 (10%)	48
Total	29	31	23	5	88

TABLE 9.2. Gender in heterosexual relationships: Disclosure of HIV status is of primary concern.

	Strongly agree	Agree	Disagree	Strongly disagree	Total
Female	6 (30%)	6 (30%)	6 (30%)	2 (10%)	20
Male	23 (34%)	25 (37%)	17 (25%)	3 (4%)	68
Total	29	31	23	5	88

TABLE 9.3. HIV-positive partners in heterosexual relationships: Disclosure of HIV status is of primary concern.

	Strongly agree	Agree	Disagree	Strongly disagree	Total
HIV-positive women	4 (40%)	6 (60%)	0	0	10
HIV-positive men	5 (50%)	5 (50%)	0	0	10
HIV-negative women	6 (60%)	0	4 (40%)	0	10
HIV-negative men	6 (60%)	4 (40%)	0	0	10
Total	21	15	4	0	40

serodiscordant relationships tends to seek social support more than the male, and that when the female is HIV negative she is more likely to disclose to family than when she is HIV positive.

African-American and Hispanic partners in serodiscordant couples reported the highest level of distress from disclosure issues (Table 9.4). When collapsing strongly agree with agree categories, an overwhelming 86 percent of Hispanics reported that disclosing HIV status was a primary concern in their relationship. Among those who identified themselves as white, only 43 percent reported disclosure as a primary issue in their relationship. This was an anticipated finding given the intense cultural and religious proscription against homosexuality that has continued to make it difficult to disclose an HIV diagnosis to one's family and friends in the community (Marks et al., 1992). So again, the numerous tiers for clinical work with a couple affected by HIV must include sensitivity to the cultural and religious variables that some partners and couples may share, always remembering that great diversity exists within each culture that is informed by the uniqueness of each relationship and each partner. Helping HIV-affected couples deal with disclosing their HIV diagnosis must include attention to how their families of origin have integrated the many different values and norms espoused by their religious, cultural, and regional norms about the meaning of illness, and the particular emotional reactions to HIV/AIDS.

Interestingly, less than a quarter (20 percent) of HIV-positive partners strongly agreed that disclosure was of primary concern in their relationship while nearly half (45.5 percent) of HIV-negative partners strongly agreed that it was a primary concern (Table 9.5). As Walker (1991) explains, though HIV affects both partners, the HIV-negative partner is routinely excluded from the medical model and therefore is without formal structural support. Narrative responses and case summaries support and explain this finding as they illustrate that the HIV-negative partner often prefers to disclose sooner and to more people to gain emotional support and acknowledgment. The HIV-negative

TABLE 9.4. Ethnicity: Disclosure of HIV status is of primary concern.

	Strongly agree	Agree	Disagree	Strongly disagree	Total
African American	13 (57%)	7 (30%)	2 (9%)	1 (4%)	23
Hispanic	11 (39%)	13 (46%)	3 (11%)	1 (4%)	28
White	5 (13%)	11 (30%)	18 (49%)	3 (8%)	37
Total	29	31	23	5	88

TABLE 9.5. Serostatus: Disclosure of HIV status is of primary concern.

	Strongly agree	Agree	Disagree	Strongly disagree	Total
HIV positive	9 (20%)	15 (34.5%)	15 (34.5%)	5 (11%)	44
HIV negative	20 (45.5%)	16 (36.5%)	8 (18%)	0	44
Total	29	31	23	5	88

partner may feel unattended to in the typical service provision of AIDS service organizations, and therefore is eager to be reassured by family and friends as they try to cope with their emotional reactions to how HIV has changed their lives.

The majority (63 percent) of those partners that had been together less than five years strongly agreed that HIV disclosure to others was a primary concern, whereas only 10 percent of those who had been together longer strongly agreed. In fact, 30 percent of longer-term couples disagreed that HIV disclosure to others was an area of concern in their relationship. Again, this speaks to the stability and resilience more commonly found in longer-term relationships. In general, the longer partners have been together, the less distressed they appear by these HIV-related challenges, and this has been consistent throughout this study and is seen in Table 9.6.

Those couples who were both aware of the HIV diagnosis before the relationship became serious fared better with the issue of disclosure than those who learned of the HIV diagnosis after they were an established couple. As seen in Table 9.7, less than 10 percent of those couples diagnosed before the relationship strongly identified disclosure as a source of relationship distress, whereas 46 percent of the couples who learned of the HIV diagnosis later in the relationship perceived the issue of disclosure to be problematic for them as a couple.

Couples who have experienced an HIV-related illness appear to have less concern about HIV disclosure. This seems to be self-evident as once a partner has been ill, the couple has other concerns more primary than who to tell and when. Often, the first illness is the catalyst for a disclosure process that may start at the workplace of the

TABLE 9.6. Length of relationship: Disclosure of HIV status is of primary concern.

	Strongly agree	Agree	Disagree	Strongly disagree	Total
Less than 5 years	24 (63%)	6 (16%)	8 (21%)	0	38
More than 5 years	5 (10%)	25 (50%)	15 (30%)	5 (10%)	50
Total	29	31	23	5	88

TABLE 9.7. When couple learned of HIV diagnosis: Disclosure of HIV status is of primary concern.

	Strongly agree	Agree	Disagree	Strongly disagree	Total
Diagnosed before relationship	3 (9%)	11 (34%)	14 (44%)	4 (13%)	32
Diagnosed in relationship	26 (46%)	20 (36%)	9 (16%)	1 (2%)	56
Total	29	31	23	5	88

TABLE 9.8. HIV-related illness: Disclosure of HIV status is of primary concern.

	Strongly agree	Agree	Disagree	Strongly disagree	Total
Have had HIV illness	11 (21%)	15 (29%)	21 (40%)	5 (10%)	52
Have not had HIV illness	18 (50%)	16 (44%)	2 (6%)	0	36
Total	29	31	23	5	88

HIV-positive partner and move on to include the family and friends both partners were avoiding telling. This supposition is supported by the fact that 40 percent of those who have experienced HIV-related illness disagreed that disclosure was a primary concern. Compare this with the 5 percent of those who have not had an HIV-related illness who strongly disagreed that disclosure was a primary issue for them as seen in Table 9.8.

QUALITATIVE FINDINGS

Narrative Responses

When respondents commented on how conflict over HIV disclosure has manifested in their relationships, two distinct disclosure issues emerged. The most common set of narrative responses revolved around the HIV-negative partner wanting to disclose his or her partner's HIV status to family and friends whereas the HIV-positive partner did not. The other complexity surrounding disclosure was that by "coming out" with HIV, the HIV-positive partner is coming out as gay or as a recent injection drug user to those outside of the relationship. This was more of an individual dilemma for HIV-positive men who have not "come out" to their families as gay men than representative of a dyadic conflict in the relationship. Examples of both are provided as follows.

Conflicting Wishes About Disclosing HIV Status to Others

"I just assumed we'd tell both families about his diagnosis, but he doesn't want to and doesn't want me to tell my family either."

"I don't want to tell my parents and this causes us a lot of tension because he feels we should tell them."

"I hate that this is a secret. I want to tell my family and friends and he feels we shouldn't until we have to."

"I want to tell more of our friends, but he seems afraid to or ashamed to. But I can't really tell them because it's his diagnosis, his news. I have to wait until he's ready."

"We've been fighting about this a lot because I don't want to keep her diagnosis secret, but she does. It puts me in a really awkward situation. I feel like I'm lying to people by not telling them what we're living with."

"We know we should tell our families, but I think they'd be too upset. He pressures me to just do it and get it over with, but he doesn't realize how upset and frightened they would be. I'm their only son."

"We've already been rejected by my family, I don't want to risk that again."

Disclosing More Than HIV Status

"If it were just the HIV diagnosis, I think I could do it, but it isn't. They'll put two and two together and realize that I'm gay and Rob is my boyfriend."

"He's more concerned about his parents than me. He'd rather keep them in the dark about us than stand up for me and our relationship."

"My husband never told his family about his drug use. If we tell them about his diagnosis, they're going to think he's gay or a drug user and we wouldn't want to have that conversation."

"We were able to tell our immediate families, but they asked us not to tell anybody else. Y'know cousins and stuff still don't know I'm gay."

"I don't want my wife's friends and families feeling sorry for me or trying to figure out how I got it. We just deal with it on our own."

Case Studies

Case I: Mike and Claude

Mike and Claude are a couple who were discussed in Chapter 7 who had sustained a stable emotional intimacy and then experienced "drifting apart" after the HIV diagnosis. This is a couple who met during their teen years and established a close friendship that evolved into a relationship in their early twenties. They decided to start a family and adopt a child and both were tested "just to make sure" neither was infected. They both felt confident they would test negative; however, Mike tested HIV positive.

There was a period of acute shock, which lasted for several weeks. While Claude seemed to carry all the anxiety for the couple, Mike responded with depression. In addition to coping with the reality of the diagnosis, Mike and Claude also argued about disclosing Mike's HIV status as Claude wanted to be able to tell his mother and family and Mike did not want anybody to know he had tested positive.

This is consistent with their positioning within their families of origin as Mike experienced great conflict coming out as a gay man to his family and Claude and his mother "shared everything." Now, as a couple living with Mike's HIV diagnosis, holding on to their respective patterns created a no-win power struggle. The following transcript highlights the exposition of this conflict.

MIKE: Look, it's my diagnosis and my family and I know they can't deal with it. I can't tell them.

CLAUDE: You don't know that. You never tried. And now, it's like we're gonna have to keep this secret forever. I just can't.

MIKE: What do you mean you can't? It's not for you to do.

CLAUDE: Well, what are we gonna do? Wait for you to get sick and then I'm gonna have to tell them?

According to Mike and Claude, this was a fight they have had repeatedly since couple therapy had moved them past fighting about the dishes. This was one of their "big issues" they had avoided before couple therapy. Although they did disclose to several friends, it was always Claude (the HIV-negative partner) pushing to disclose Mike's positive result and Mike always resisting disclosing. Both partners remained inflexible regarding Mike's family. As with other issues in this relationship, Claude's anxiety pushed him into the pursuer role, and in response, Mike became more distant and more obstinate. This is a dynamic that may take place with any couple around any issue, but for Mike and Claude it emerged around HIV disclosure.

Although other approaches were used with this couple, emotionally focused couple therapy was used with Mike and Claude to de-escalate their pattern and understand their positioning with this issue. From this approach, the aim would also include helping Mike and Claude to step out of their rigid positions and expand their emotional responses. By doing so, the interactional dynamic will be shifted. As Johnson and Williams-Keeler (1998) said, "[W]hen a previously hostile partner touches and expresses his or her fear . . . confiding and compassion may begin" (p. 451). The behavioral positioning is a manifestation of the underlying emotional experiences of each partner, now complicated by the HIV diagnosis and all that that may entail in their conscious and unconscious processes. In order to restructure their positioning around this standoff they must be helped to understand the need to take such a position, the underlying anxieties about disclosing or not disclosing the diagnosis. The first broad task then is to facilitate a safe environment for them to express core emotional experiences that fuel their respective positioning.

THERAPIST: Clearly, you both feel strongly about this and your conversations so far haven't provided either of you with relief or resolution. Let's put aside what you will or won't do for now. Let's try to work together on getting a better grip on what telling Mike's family means for both of you.

MIKE: I know my mother. I know she'll be devastated. It'll break her heart and I can't do it.

THERAPIST: So for you Mike, one concern is that you feel like you have to protect your mom?

MIKE: Yeah. She's getting older. She lost my dad. She doesn't do well with stress and I guess I'm just hoping I don't have to tell her.

THERAPIST: Claude, what do you hear about what Mike is going through about telling people?

CLAUDE: He's afraid to tell his mother. I know that, but, y'know, she will live and she will get over it and I think. . . . [Mike is rolling his eyes.]

THERAPIST: I'm going to ask you guys to avoid solving this right now and focus more or making yourself understood or understanding what it is you're feeling about this.

CLAUDE: I understand you feel afraid to tell your mother. I do understand about her. But do you understand that this is bigger than your mother. You're asking me to keep this a secret from my family and some of our friends? I don't think that's fair.

THERAPIST: [Trying to elicit less anger and frustration and prime Claude to articulate more of his other vulnerable feelings that Mike may be able to relate to.] So you're frustrated in part that Mike seems to be calling the shots, but it sounds like you're also feeling some other things about not being able to share this news with other people in your life. Is that right?

CLAUDE: I'm all alone with this. He's tied my hands because he doesn't want too many of our friends to know and it makes me feel like I can't talk to anyone about it. He talks to his doctor every month and the other people at the clinic. I'm like . . . "just watching" like I'm not living with this also.

In reflecting the many subtleties that occur in this dynamic, both partners are helped to better understand how their underlying emotions (largely anxiety and isolation) have created an obstruction in their ability to hear each other or relate to each other. In addition, as they perpetuate an "attack-attack" dynamic, communication becomes fully obstructed.

This attack-attack interaction was reflected as problematic, and although some immediate attention focused on communication improvements in terms of how they talked about disclosing, the emphasis remained on facilitating an emotional reengagement between Mike and Claude. This was met with a powerful undertow by their system as they tried to hold onto this dynamic and power struggle about disclosure. By not colluding with either partner, or colluding in maintaining this as an irresoluble conflict on a behavioral plane, work was able to fluctuate between their underlying emotions and their behavioral positioning. When the empathic connection was reestablished, they were very ready to develop a more adaptive way of resolving the action component of who to tell and when.

THERAPIST: So when Mike says he wants to keep his diagnosis very private, are you able to understand what it means for him? How he feels about it?

CLAUDE: I guess. It's still kind of foreign to me that this would happen and he wouldn't tell his family. . . . I mean in my family. . . .

THERAPIST: I know it's very different from how you would like to deal with it . . . but are you able to understand how it makes him feel to keep it to himself, even from his family?

CLAUDE: I guess like he holds the power of when he'll tell. That he wants it to be up to him, when he feels ready.

MIKE: Is that so bad? I just feel like all our decisions have been taken away from us since this happened. This is one thing . . . I can still decide . . . because once I tell people I can't undo it. They'll always see me like this, and think about me with this, and see me getting sick. I just don't want to deal with it. . . . I don't want to have to deal with it. I don't know if I can see this in everybody's eyes . . . [becomes very sad and teary].

CLAUDE: [Covers Mike's hand with his own.] Okay. Okay. [Long quiet during which they are holding hands as Mike pulls himself together and is comforted by Claude.]

MIKE: Listen, I understand you have a right to talk to your friends and family too. I don't want you to feel alone about this. I just don't want to tell my mother, not yet. . . . just don't think I can face it. Maybe if we could talk about who you'd tell first, I'd feel better.

At the heart of EFCT is the premise that emotion "is determinant of attachment behavior" and can be used as a primary tool in shifting maladaptive interactional positions, such as the standoff regarding HIV disclosure between Mike and Claude. As Johnson and Williams-Keeler (1998) explain, emotions in the room, whether emanating from intrapsychic or interpersonal triggers, should not be contained or overcome, but rather understood and, if possible, felt by both partners in order to enhance their emotional engagement, which will in turn enhance their behavioral positioning with each other.

As some of the underlying emotions of Mike and Claude were elicited, and each was helped to remain focused on understanding each other's emotions, their empathic bond around this issue was shored up and renewed. This enabled us to move onto and through later stages and tasks of EFCT, such as gaining deeper insight about the nature of their attachment to each other and their families of origin, and how conflict around disclosure manifested underlying attachment issues for both Mike and Claude. With dyadic facilitation (helping them to talk directly to each other) and dyadic interpretation (having them use the therapist as an interpreter, with each talking to the therapist first and the therapist explaining to the listening partner what was said in a way he may be able to relate to it), we explored how the disclosure conflict manifested underlying attachment needs and issues.

Mike experienced a fear of abandonment from his mother and was worried that when she found out about his diagnosis, he might be shunned by her and his family of origin. He had also been uncomfortable with feelings of dependency and he feared that by disclosing his HIV status to his family he could lose some of his independence. He was experiencing dueling fears: one that his family would abandon him if he disclosed that he was HIV positive, and the other that he would be engulfed by them in ways that would make him feel embarrassed or dependent.

THERAPIST: [To Mike] I sense this is really hard for you to talk about. Maybe we can start by talking about what it's been like for you to have more friends know.

MIKE: [Big sigh.] Overall, I think it's a relief and I think it's one less thing Claude and I fight about. I think it's been more helpful to him than me. I would still rather nobody know.

THERAPIST: Mike, what's it like for you that Claude has a different take on this, and obviously is rooting for you to tell your mom?

MIKE: Well, I mostly feel like that's his need. He thinks I'll feel better if I tell them, that they'll rally around me, that he'll be able to share his concerns with them. I think that's his need. Honestly, the reality is that my mother will be devastated. Devastated and angry and maybe even not be able to accept it . . . or me. . . .

CLAUDE: Well then, what are you protecting? If she's gonna turn her back on you, then why are you so worried about her?

MIKE: You don't understand. I can't do this to her. She's been through enough. It was all she could do to not keel over when I told her I was gay. Now I'm gonna tell her I have HIV. My mother will be out of her mind. My family's not like yours. They might turn their backs. I'm not sure I want to lose them.

THERAPIST: Earlier when we spoke about you not telling your mom, it felt like you were really concerned that she couldn't take this news. Now there's another level, there's also you protecting whatever tie you have with her. Is that right?

MIKE: I don't want to lose my mother and I don't want people looking at me and only seeing the HIV. It's about me and my mother and I want to be able to take care of it when I think I can.

CLAUDE: Okay. I just wish we could tell them, so you, we, don't feel so alone, but okay. I guess that's that. I won't bring it up again.

Here, Mike is asserting an autonomy and independence that he feels he has had to defend since the diagnosis. This is consistent with earlier transactions in which he explained that he did not want to become dependent on Claude or Claude's opinion about disclosure or other HIV-related matters. One can see that the underlying fear of abandonment by his mother was a primary contributor to the rigid position he took regarding disclosing to his family. For Claude, his desire to tell Mike's family comes from, in part, his wish to be part of a larger system, to feel less alone. And so, as Claude pushes for disclosure to Mike's mom (the last frontier), Mike becomes fearful and depressed. As Mike becomes fearful and depressed, Claude feels more anxious and instinctively seeks more family support. This is one example of how both partners' underlying attachment issues fueled their behavioral positioning around disclosure.

With these insights integrated, and feeling more emotionally attached to each other, they were able to shift their behaviors in relation to each other and the issues surrounding Mike's HIV disclosure. In time, they were able to integrate and consolidate more mutually satisfying resolutions to this conflict. Mike's restriction on Claude that he tell very few people of the HIV diagnosis was lifted. Claude was able to tell his mother and sister, and was met with tremendous solidarity and emotional support from both family members. This lifted his spirits and lessened some of his anxieties.

Mike struggled with wanting to tell his family, but felt too frightened to do so. He was, however, helped by Claude to tell several more friends who were all supportive to Mike individually, and to Mike and Claude as a couple of mixed HIV status. They reported feeling relieved and much closer around this issue. Unfortunately for Mike, he still was unable to confide in his family and remained sad and conflicted about it.

Case II: Gary and Tim

Gary is a twenty-five-year-old art student who tested HIV positive when he was twenty-one. Tim is a thirty-six-year-old African-American lawyer who met and "married" Gary two years ago. They quickly built a full life together, which included shared friends, shared interests and goals, and Tim's integration into Gary's family of origin as Gary's partner. They have enjoyed great satisfaction and sustained emotional intimacy. They explained that issues surrounding their serodiscordance have not created significant conflict.

The only conflict that emerged from their serodiscordance was that Tim never told his family that he is gay or that Gary is HIV positive. Tim feels his family, who are Methodist and "very religious," will never accept his homosexuality. After trying to come out to his parents and finding it too difficult, he resigned himself that he would never share his life with them truthfully.

After Gary's episode of pneumonia, they began to experience intense conflict about Tim's refusal to tell his family the truth. Each time Gary heard Tim lying to his family he became very angry and demanded that Tim "step up to the plate" on telling them that he was gay and that Gary may be ill.

This was a relationship with a strong and secure bond, but the upset of Gary's illness impaired their capacity for negotiation and resiliency around disclosure conflicts. Because each partner was anxious about Gary's illness, the focus of intervention had to be understood as intrapsychic and interpersonal or as Johnson and Williams-Keeler (1998) describe it, "within and between."

Both Gary and Tim were helped to articulate their emotional reactions to Gary's illness and for both it felt like a defining moment in their lives as a couple and, of course, as individuals. Gary felt that he could no longer condone Tim's lying or his participation in Tim's lying to his family. Tim, who had made his peace with not telling his family about his relationship with Gary, was even more afraid of disclosing Gary's HIV status. They engaged in repetitive arguments and decided to come in for a consultation.

GARY: I won't hide my life. I won't hide my relationship with you and just can't accept that you still would.

TIM: I know. I can't help it. I just can't. I wish you'd stop pressuring me.

THERAPIST: When telling people about our illnesses, people have lots of mixed feelings and different ways of handling it. Some of what you seem to be feeling with each other is clearly frustration. I'm wondering if you can help each other understand what other feelings come up for you about telling or not telling Tim's family about your life together?

GARY: Well, I can't believe he's more worried about upsetting his family than upsetting me. I mean I may be sick again. Should I be ashamed of it? Should I go along with lying about us? Either they'll get over it or they won't [turns directly to Tim], but where's your pride . . . where's your concern for me?

TIM: I know. I know you're right. But I just can't. The more you pressure me, the more paralyzed I get. Just give me a little space. What's the urgency?

THERAPIST: Tim, other than Gary wanting you to tell your family about him, what else did you hear Gary saying?

TIM: That he's put me in the middle between him and them. He's saying he feels I'm choosing to take care of them over him, but that's not true. . . .

THERAPIST: Let's hold off on what's true or not true and stay with what Gary's feelings are about this. He's looking for a different level of commitment, of security that shows that you care about him enough that your relationship not be hidden from those in your world, even in the face of possible rejection. Does that sound right Gary?

GARY: Yes. I don't mean it as a showdown, them or me, but I do feel like I shouldn't have to lie about us or my diagnosis and that I would feel more secure about us to see him stand up to his family and come out fully as a gay man with an HIV-positive partner.

TIM: I know. I need to work on this. You do come first, you know that. I need you to give me more time to figure out how I could do it. I can't stand all this fighting and all this pressure. I'm freaked out also y'know. Just give me a little space to figure it out. After what we just went through, I just want to slow down and catch our breath before creating another crisis.

THERAPIST: It seems like your needs in this relationship shifted a bit after Gary's health scare. That you had different reactions to the upset. For you Gary, it upped the ante in terms of your need to feel Tim's strength and his bond with you? And that for you Tim, it makes you feel like all you want is comfort and safety right now, not a return to your conflict about telling your family?

Both Gary and Tim were experiencing some insecurity since Gary's illness, and the result is that Gary is looking for a deeper level of commitment from Tim, and Tim is looking for stability and relief from conflict and chaos. These needs can also be understood as attachment needs. Returning to the theoretical integration of EFCT and HIV, if HIV is experienced as an attachment injury, then the first wave of illness will elicit anxiety about the security of that bond. Is it secure enough to weather further illness? Will the attachment provide the partners with safety and stability in the face of their anxieties? This push for disclosure was Gary's need to experience Tim's loyalty and protection of their relationship. What EFCT offers is the conceptualization and normalization of attachment needs such as comfort, safety, security, and dependency in an adult relationship.

In the face of illness, Gary and Tim's underlying attachment needs were activated and manifested around this standoff regarding disclosure of Tim's HIV status to his family. By fostering insight and empathic responses for both partners, they were better able to avoid the rigid positioning that resulted in a nonproductive pattern of pressure and withdrawal around disclosure. New positioning included the flexibility of providing Tim with a bit more space and room to work out his conflict and alternative demonstrations of love and commitment from Tim to Gary. Although Tim and Gary did not resolve this issue entirely, it was an issue they were much more able to discuss without destructive or distancing fighting.

SUMMARY

These were just two case examples about how disclosure may affect a couple of mixed HIV status, but so many of any couple's issues are interrelated and interdependent, and as emotional engagement was reconstructed in this area, other conflicts were diffused as well. The practitioner has to balance the simultaneous levels, individual and dyadic, of conflict HIV disclosure often activates. Each individual can be helped to cope with his or her feelings about disclosing an HIV diagnosis (or homosexuality), and each couple has to negotiate the feelings that are provoked between each other by who and when they tell people in their lives about the HIV diagnosis.

Emotionally focused couple therapy, which focuses on discovering and reorganizing the respective emotional experiences of partners, is well suited for issues of disclosure. How disclosing one's HIV status, or one's partner's HIV diagnosis to loved ones outside of the relationship can often provoke profound emotional challenges, whether the disclosure is in the workplace, extended family, or even to one's own children. Underlying attachment anxieties such as ambivalence about who can be depended on and who can't, and the natural strain between wishing for intimacy and fearing abandonment, may accompany disclosure issues for the serodiscordant couple.

Chapter 10

Issues of Mistrust and Betrayal

"I just can't trust him after this. I always worry that he's lying to me, even about the smallest thing."

OVERVIEW

With the HIV diagnosis of one partner, more than 20 percent of couples reported that broken trust and feelings of betrayal were a primary concern in their relationship. Two distinct injuries to trust emerged. Many of these feelings of betrayal emanated from the way and when a couple learns of their serodiscordance. The first scenario of betrayal occurred when couples had been dating for some time with the assumption of shared HIV-negative status until one partner confided that they were HIV positive.

Whatever foundation of trust has been enjoyed in the early stages of the relationship may be seriously injured or even destroyed. Mancilla and Troshinsky (2003) reported an increasing pattern of new couples getting tested earlier than later as a "rite of passage to trust" (p. 73).

In the other scenario of HIV and broken trust, a positive HIV test is the evidence of a broken contract between partners, an affair in which there was unprotected sexual activity. Even for couples who have a nonmonogamous relationship, there may be a violation of a pact to maintain safer sex practices in any relationships outside of theirs. This can result in a profound experience of betrayal that mars the sense of trust and good faith between partners and may threaten the survival of the relationship or be a lingering and serious injury to the couple's life together. The individual experiences of how trust is broken by learning of the serodiscordance are expanded on in detail in narrative comments from respondents and case studies later in this chapter.

QUANTITATIVE FINDINGS

Findings confirm that issues of mistrust and betrayal are common but not central to this sample of serodiscordant couples. Regarding sexual orientation, noteworthy differences were seen in the extent mistrust was related to a couple's serodiscordance (Table 10.1). Feelings and issues surrounding mistrust and betrayal were more common among heterosexual couples, with 32.5 percent of heterosexuals strongly agreeing that mistrust and betrayal due to the HIV diagnosis is a primary concern in their relationship, whereas only 12.5 percent of gay male couples strongly agreed that this was of primary concern. In fact, gay couples felt so strongly that the HIV diagnosis was not associated with betrayal that 68.5 percent disagreed, whereas only 30 percent of heterosexual couples disagreed. This may be explained by somewhat different norms between heterosexual and gay male couples regarding dating and relationships, with gay male relationships somewhat more flexible in allowing for variations on a strictly monogamous contract (Mancilla and Troshinsky, 2003). In addition, it is more normative and anticipated to have a conversation about serostatus among gay males than among heterosexual couples as courtships begin (Mancilla and Troshinsky, 2003).

Women tended to experience many more concerns regarding broken trust than their male counterparts (Table 10.2). In fact, 55 percent of females strongly agreed, whereas only 12 percent of males agreed that betrayal became a primary issue when a partner was diagnosed

TABLE 10.1. Sexual orientation: Mistrust/betrayal is of primary concern.

	Strongly agree	Agree	Disagree	Strongly disagree	Total
Heterosexual	13 (32.5%)	15 (37.5%)	8 (20%)	4 (10%)	40
Homosexual	6 (12.5%)	9 (19%)	15 (31%)	18 (37.5%)	48
Total	19	24	23	22	88

with HIV. This is partially explained by the higher rates of mistrust and betrayal within heterosexual relationships. Of course, gender norms are also a component, with women traditionally socialized to experience and to express more vulnerability than males (Greenan and Tunnell, 2003).

Not surprisingly, partners who are HIV negative in heterosexual relationships reported that issues of mistrust and betrayal were more of a primary concern than their HIV-positive partners (Table 10.3). Whether couples go through the broken trust early or later in the relation-

TABLE 10.2. Gender in heterosexual relationships: Mistrust/betrayal is of primary concern.

	Strongly agree	Agree	Disagree	Strongly disagree	Total
Female	11 (55%)	5 (25%)	2 (10%)	2 (10%)	20
Male	8 (12%)	19 (28%)	21 (31%)	20 (29%)	68
Total	19	24	23	22	88

TABLE 10.3. HIV-positive partners in heterosexual relationships: Mistrust/betrayal is of primary concern.

	Strongly agree	Agree	Disagree	Strongly disagree	Total
HIV-positive women	0	2 (20%)	6 (60%)	2 (20%)	10
HIV-positive men	0	8 (80%)	2 (20%)	0	10
HIV-negative women	6 (60%)	4 (40%)	0	0	10
HIV-negative men	7 (70%)	1 (10%)	0	2 (20%)	10
Total	13	15	8	4	40

ship, HIV-negative partners tended to feel more betrayed by the news of an HIV diagnosis in their relationship.

Little or no notable differences existed among different ethnicities in so many of the issues that emerged for serodiscordant couples (Table 10.4). However, in examining the issue of how HIV has created mistrust and betrayal in relationships, significantly different experiences were reported. The rates were significantly higher among African Americans, with 44 percent identifying betrayal as a primary issue. For Hispanic couples, 25 percent of the sample reported this as a primary concern in their relationship. Only 5 percent of white respondents reported betrayal as a primary issue. This may be explained by particularly strong cultural and religious taboos within African-American and Hispanic cultures related to extramarital affairs and bisexual or homosexual orientations.

Regardless of sexual orientation, HIV-negative partners in serodiscordant relationships reported that issues of mistrust and betrayal were more of a primary concern than did their HIV-positive partners (Table 10.5). Once mistrust is experienced by the HIV-negative partner, it remains a struggle for the couple.

Unfortunately, the study is unable to determine how the couple learned of their serodiscordance, and so the most that can be determined is that couples that were more newly formed had many more issues of mistrust and betrayal around their serodiscordance than longer-term couples (Table 10.6). In fact, when collapsing the two agree categories, 76 percent agreed that mistrust and betrayal was an issue

TABLE 10.4. Ethnicity: Mistrust/betrayal is of primary concern.

	Strongly agree	Agree	Disagree	Strongly disagree	Total
African American	10 (44%)	8 (35%)	4 (17%)	1 (4%)	23
Hispanic	7 (25%)	8 (29%)	9 (32%)	4 (14%)	28
White	2 (5%)	8 (22%)	10 (27%)	17 (46%)	37
Total	19	24	23	22	88

of primary concern, whereas only 28 percent of longer-term couples identified mistrust and betrayal as a primary concern.

Concurring with recent literature on how couples cope with sero-discordance, partners who revealed their positive HIV status during friendship or dating stage experienced significantly less distress with issues of betrayal (Mancilla and Troshinsky, 2003) (Table 10.7). The sooner a couple is aware of their difference in HIV status, the less mistrust and betrayal will arise between partners. Those partners who knew of their serodiscordance before they identified themselves as a couple fared much better. With no respondent strongly agreeing that mixed HIV status caused mistrust and betrayal, categories of strongly agree and agree are collapsed. The significant difference is highlighted between those couples who knew of their different HIV status before the relationship was formed, and those couples who learned of their serodiscordance after they were an established couple as seen in Table 10.7.

TABLE 10.5. Serostatus: Mistrust/betrayal is of primary concern.

	Strongly agree	Agree	Disagree	Strongly disagree	Total
HIV positive	3 (7%)	9 (20%)	14 (32%)	18 (41%)	44
HIV negative	16 (36%)	15 (34%)	9 (20%)	4 (10%)	44
Total	19	24	23	22	88

TABLE 10.6. Length of relationship: Mistrust/betrayal is of primary concern.

	Strongly agree	Agree	Disagree	Strongly disagree	Total
Less than 5 years	14 (37%)	15 (39%)	5 (13%)	4 (11%)	38
More than 5 years	5 (10%)	9 (18%)	18 (36%)	18 (36%)	50
Total	19	24	23	22	88

The experience of an HIV-related illness does not appear to influence the degree to which feelings of mistrust/betrayal present as a concern for serodiscordant couples (Table 10.8). Twenty-nine percent of those couples who had lived through an illness reported issues of mistrust/betrayal. Of those couples who had not experienced an HIV-related illness, 11 percent reported similarly that they had been coping with issues of mistrust/betrayal in their relationship.

QUALITATIVE FINDINGS

Narrative Responses

Feelings of mistrust and betrayal as they related to serodiscordance were found under two circumstances. The first situation that provokes high levels of mistrust and betrayal occurs during courtship. If

TABLE 10.7. When couple learned of HIV diagnosis: Mistrust/betrayal is of primary concern.

	Strongly agree	Agree	Disagree	Strongly disagree	Total
Diagnosed before relationship	0	9 (28%)	13 (41%)	10 (31%)	32
Diagnosed in relationship	19 (34%)	15 (27%)	10 (18%)	12 (21%)	56
Total	19	24	23	22	88

TABLE 10.8. HIV-related illness: Mistrust/betrayal is of primary concern.

	Strongly agree	Agree	Disagree	Strongly disagree	Total
Have had HIV illness	15 (29%)	13 (25%)	13 (25%)	11 (21%)	52
Have not had HIV illness	4 (11%)	11 (30%)	10 (28%)	11 (31%)	36
Total	19	24	23	22	88

a dating partner is HIV positive and does not share this with his or her boyfriend or girlfriend while they are becoming serious and attached to each other, there is a likelihood that the HIV-negative partner will feel betrayed when this news is shared later on. For long-term couples that have shared HIV-negative status, there is usually some form of understanding about staying HIV negative. Perhaps they have entered into an explicit marital contract or commitment ceremony that signifies monogamy. Perhaps they have an understanding that nonmonogamy is allowed as long as each partner practices safer sex. Whatever the unique understanding between partners is, it usually does not include bringing HIV into their relationship. Narrative responses to open-ended questions highlight and confirm these experiences.

Mistrust/Betrayal That Occurs During Dating

"I think I still doubt him sometimes and it goes back to the beginning with all the secrets. He didn't tell me he was positive until we were already falling in love. I felt like he lied to me from the beginning."

"The foundation of trust between us was shaky from the start. She never got over that I didn't tell her earlier about my HIV status. Now she thinks I'm withholding other stuff. I guess I didn't trust that she would still want to be with me after I told her."

"I can't blame her for always being suspicious. I should have been forthcoming about my status from the beginning."

"I know she was afraid to tell me, but it's like she waited so long that when she told me, I really felt betrayed. How could she keep that from me?"

Mistrust/Betrayal That Occurs Due to Break in Agreement Between Partners

"Honestly, I can never trust him again. Not only was he acting out, but actually contracted the virus and brought it into our relationship, our life, our future. . . . I don't think I can ever forgive him."

"I knew my husband was probably having sex outside the relationship, but I thought he'd protect himself at least. Everything's different now. Not to mention I don't know where he got the virus from."

"I worry that he's been doin' this all along and now maybe he infected me. Maybe I'll show up with the virus or something because he was screwing around. It's hard to get over that."

"I thought he was monogamous with me. I was with him. He's acting out all over the place and I feel like a fool for trusting him. Never again."

"I know I lost his trust. I don't know what I can ever do to win his respect back."

Case Studies

Case I: Nicole and James

Nicole is a thirty-five-year-old African-American woman who has overcome a chaotic childhood and family life marked by many different men in her mother's life and many moves to different neighborhoods and different schools. She has worked as a secretary most of her adult life, but has never moved out of her mother's home and has had numerous addictive episodes through her teen years. She was able to break the addictive cycle with injection drugs and alcohol and had been hopeful in recent years about settling down with her long-term boyfriend.

During her pregnancy almost two years ago, she was tested for HIV and learned that she had contracted the virus. Nicole's boyfriend, the father of their baby, left her when she told him that she was HIV positive. She told her sister and her mother, who both reacted with fear and anxiety about her health. They expressed alarm as to what might occur if extended family and community members found out that Nicole had HIV. Nicole felt she needed to keep her diagnosis secret at all costs to protect herself and her family.

Several months after she found out about her diagnosis, she began seeing James, a friend from the neighborhood. Much to her surprise, James turned out to be "a really good guy" who she felt very safe with and close to. As their relationship began forming, she struggled for months with conflicted feelings about telling him that she was HIV positive. Although she intended to tell him, she felt unable to take the risk that he would break up with her if he knew she was HIV positive.

James, a thirty-one-year-old African-American man from Nicole's neighborhood, worked in a hospital as a clerk. He came from a large religious family in which he was the youngest sibling. His mother died suddenly from a heart attack when he was eleven years old. His father worked two jobs and was never around. In many ways he felt he raised himself after his mother died. He describes himself as a "loner" who had difficulty making friends. He had only one previous girlfriend before Nicole and that relationship ended abruptly when his girlfriend left him for her ex-boyfriend.

From a casual friendship, Nicole and James were drawn to each other and the relationship became romantic. James was integrated quickly into Nicole's family and life. He helped her take care of her baby and made her feel she could depend on him for financial and emotional support. For both partners, they described this relationship as a happiness they hadn't expected to experience. Through ten months of dating, Nicole tried to tell James of her HIV status but couldn't. James ultimately found out through Nicole's sister when she inadvertently asked how he was holding up with the extra stress of Nicole's health problems.

James was stunned and felt betrayed by Nicole. He was very seriously considering breaking up with Nicole, not because she was HIV positive, but because she didn't tell him that she was.

This couple was seen for several sessions and it was instantly clear that they were at cross-purposes. James indicated he thought the relationship could not survive this break in trust and he wanted help breaking up with her. Nicole desperately wanted to be forgiven and to have a second chance to renew his faith in her.

JAMES: I don't even know why I'm here. We can't work anything out.

NICOLE: Let's just try and see if she can help us [pleading with James].

THERAPIST: Can you tell me what you hope to get out of us meeting?

NICOLE: We've been together for almost a year. It's been really great. I want to save this relationship. James is a good man, and I let him down. I just don't know how many times I can apologize. He won't forgive me.

THERAPIST: [Trying to engage James] Can either of you tell me what's been happening?

NICOLE: I should've told him I had the virus. I was going to, but I just was so scared that if I told him, he'd leave me.

THERAPIST: James? What's this been like for you?

JAMES: Maybe she's sorry, but I don't really want to be here talking about it. It happened and I just can't see anything good coming out of it anymore.

NICOLE: And that's it! You're gonna leave now. You were gonna leave either way, weren't you?

In those early minutes of this first meeting, the largest obstacle was that James barely had enough motivation to sit through the consultation. Returning to Ripple's (1964) tripartite assessment paradigm of motivation, capacity, and opportunity, this was a couple that presented numerous obstacles regarding all three resources. Whenever a partner expresses a desire to break up in a first consultation session, the therapist has to remain cognizant that whatever motivation brought him or her to session must be aggressively nourished in order to engage him or her with the therapist and the therapeutic process (if he or she is not able to engage with the partner). The presenting issue did not lend itself to identifying repetitive interactional behaviors that created dysfunction between them. Nor were they capable of building an empathic alliance with each other at this time. Several attempts were made about trying to understand how their partner experienced this episode, but intervention exploded with high emotional reactivity on both parts. With James' motivation so low, and their trust in each other devastated, the first order of business was simply engaging them as a couple with this process. With such a task, structural therapy provided the framework and the tools.

Before hypotheses could be formulated about whether this couple could or *should* survive the break in trust, a great deal of joining had to occur. As Minuchin (1984) stated, it is necessary to enter into their transactional field; to join empathetically with each partner and the couple as a unit. Extra efforts toward joining with James were made early and often in this first session. Once that was established, structural concerns regarding the couple's boundaries, homeostasis, and power seemed to present themselves.

THERAPIST: James, I hear that you don't want to be here in the worst way. That you're still very mad and hurt. I think whatever was good about the last ten months, must have been pretty good, to get you [to] come here tonight. That must've taken a lot of strength. Can you tell me a little about how things were before this happened? [This intervention assesses how they negotiated their issues and positions with one another before the crisis.]

JAMES: I don't know. I think we got along good. I really like being around her and the baby. I still can't believe this all happened.

THERAPIST: It's shocking. Maybe we can use some of the time here tonight to talk about what it's been like to find this out when you did. And, Nicole, it must be pretty overwhelming to see James so angry. It took a lot of determination to drag him here tonight. You must be kind of shocked yourself that everything happened the way it did.

NICOLE: I am. I can't believe this all blew up this way.

THERAPIST: So, you're both shocked right now. It's like this all got out of hand for you as individuals and as the couple you were just a few weeks ago.

These joining efforts and others began to shift the tenor in the room somewhat and James reluctantly became engaged with the process of trying to understand how Nicole's not telling him of her HIV status affected him. The more they spoke, the more concepts and principles from crisis intervention seemed relevant.

This couple had suffered a hazardous event (not the HIV itself, but the disclosing of the HIV after the fact that broke his trust) and were still very much in acute crisis.

Their respective norms in the relationships appeared to maintain a healthy homeostasis before the diagnosis came out. On closer examination, James had been cautious about "giving his heart" to anyone and maintained a boundary around himself that had been at times impermeable to Nicole. Sensing this, Nicole feared telling him she was HIV positive would end their relationship. In a desperate attempt to keep him, she withheld telling him and he felt betrayed. Their respective roles from their childhood were replicated in this dynamic; she as an abandoned victim and he as the betrayed loner. Not the HIV diagnosis, but the psychic injury of betrayal James experienced shattered how they had maintained their previous emotional and functional structures.

Psychodynamically, each partner had experienced numerous betrayals in their families of origin, and in some ways this left both emotionally scarred regarding basic trust.

Nicole's denial may have helped her survive in an abusive home and neighborhood, but in this instance it was maladaptive, as it resulted in the damaging of what appeared to be the "first good thing" in her life. James' impulse to withdraw may have served him well in the chaos that surrounded him in his early family life, but if this was an otherwise healthy and satisfying relationship, it may not be in his best interest to revert to his defensive posture and withdraw completely.

By the end of the first session, they both appeared engaged in the process (Nicole more than James), but they agreed to have several sessions. They were going to keep some distance and try not to work this out or break up before the next session. Internal and external resources were discussed that might provide each with support during this crisis.

In the second session, each partner chose to speak only to me (dyadic interpretation) and I rephrased their comments so that it still accurately represented their concerns about betrayal, but could be more easily taken in by their partner. This was quite helpful initially, but cannot be solely relied on as direct interaction between James and Nicole had to occur for them to learn of their typical transactional patterns (emotional and behavioral positioning with each other) and improve maladaptive transactional patterns. Structural theory posits that in-session interactions are a microcosm for patterns outside of the treatment room and make evident the unique role of norms, rules, homeostasis, and other structural dynamics of each particular couple. A brief excerpt here highlights the maladaptive pattern and the therapist's interventions to challenge and shift them.

NICOLE: I just can't apologize anymore. I don't know what else I can say to explain my behavior. At this point, you can either forgive me or you can't.

THERAPIST: How do you fight about this at home? [Fostering an enactment]

NICOLE: It's the same thing. He's never satisfied. It just goes on and on.

THERAPIST: James, can you show me how you talk about this at home?

JAMES: Yeah. It ain't me that's the problem. She doesn't seem to realize how big she screwed up. She says she's sorry, but she doesn't seem to realize she was lying to me all this time. Every time we were together. This is not the sort of thing you can just say you're sorry for and move on.

NICOLE: [Enraged] I said I'm sorry a million times, you baby! What the fuck do you want from me?

THERAPIST: Whoa. Let's get a grip here. Nicole, maybe you fight this way at home, but I'm going to ask both of you not to curse at each other and not to talk in ways that are demeaning to each other. You can say how you're feeling and curse about how you feel, but I don't want any name-calling. It just shuts us down. Here's how we'll work it, each of you can tell the other person how you feel or what you want, but you can't accuse each other.

JAMES: I want you to apologize like you mean it. I feel really hurt. I feel like a fool. Tell me you'll never lie to me again. Tell me I can trust you.

NICOLE: [In anger] I told you! I couldn't help it! You didn't get the virus. I didn't tell you . . . because I was afraid you'd leave me if you knew.

JAMES: Well, after all I've been doing for you and the baby, giving you money, checking in on your mother, helping around the house, I just thought . . . I just think . . . if it were me . . . I wouldn't have been able to keep that from you. I would've found some way. I just feel, like you don't respect me . . . or you would've told me. Whatever. That's all I'm trying to say.

Just this small excerpt highlights several structural dynamics. This couple revealed a surprising power hierarchy. Nicole appeared to be holding a great deal of the power, with James busy trying to win her over, help her with her family and financial responsibilities. The betrayal shifted the power in the relationship as James now was more powerful, threatening to leave Nicole. Further, the relative stability they enjoyed before the HIV diagnosis was apparently based on complementary roles in which James overfunctioned and Nicole underfunctioned. The way they maintained their relationship (homeostasis) was for James to compensate for Nicole in functional role demands, and it seemed he was expected not to confront or contradict her.

Although this work was condensed into several sessions, joining and enactment gave way to the third stage of structural work with couples: unbalancing. With Nicole and James demonstrating engagement and trust in the process, I was able to reflect their recurrent behavioral patterns, always making sure each partner felt heard and validated. Their typical interactional pattern perpetuated the issues of mistrust and betrayal by one of them always showing up late, taking a cell phone call while in session, etc.

The essence of the work included repair of the betrayal and facilitating more equity in the way they experienced and expressed power in the relationship. At first when James asked for Nicole's remorse, she often became defensive and hostile. He withdrew in response, and then she became angrier. By the fourth session, the pattern had shifted, with James needing to see less remorse, and Nicole feeling less accused. We were able to look at how different forms of power fueled their feelings of mistrust and betrayal.

THERAPIST: I notice that when Nicole raises her voice, you kind of get smaller James. How do you feel when she gets angry?

JAMES: I get frustrated. I feel like she just doesn't understand what I'm trying to say. I guess I give up. I always let [Nicole] win. I always let [her] have the last word.

THERAPIST: What if you changed the way you talked about this. What if, Nicole, you didn't call him any names like we've talked about and tried to just listen even if you feel upset or disagree?

JAMES: I know I wouldn't feel so disrespected.

THERAPIST: If he doesn't feel so disrespected, he doesn't need to hound you to get respect. He could more easily trust that what you feel about him is good, and that you didn't take any of this lightly or for granted. This might be the very beginning of working toward a time when he feels validated and you feel released for not being able to tell him sooner.

They were both able to moderate the way they brought this conflict up with each other, and after four sessions, they didn't return. In the last session, they were able to move into some of the underlying emotional experiences that were provoked by this break in trust. James felt he had never truly trusted anyone prior to Nicole, and this betrayal felt intolerable and seemed to be vindication for his lifelong doubts about relying on other people. Many other complexities from his childhood and family of origin, such as loss of his mother and abandonment, may have been related to the HIV diagnosis itself, but the short-term nature of therapy prevented that exploration. For Nicole, there were also issues of abandonment. Having very insecure attachments through childhood and adulthood, she was left believing that she was destined for future abandonment. Some of her behaviors with James may have set this up and confirmed her inner experiences and beliefs about the precarious nature of becoming attached to others.

Case II: Kevin and Anthony

To refresh the reader, Kevin and Anthony are a couple discussed earlier regarding their fear of HIV transmission and the impact of uncertainty exacerbated by Kevin's HIV diagnosis (a result of an extra-relationship affair).

Mistrust and betrayal between Kevin and Anthony had been a major stumbling block from its inception. The betrayal experienced by Kevin's HIV diagnosis may well have been the painful culmination of this chronic issue.

ANTHONY: I know I shouldn't bring this up . . . but we did have an understanding and Kevin's diagnosis is a constant reminder that he just totally stepped out on me and our agreement. It makes it difficult to work in good faith, because I feel like I can't trust the things he says in here.

KEVIN: I don't know what else to say. I mean you've had sex outside of the relationship. You know, on the phone, and the Internet, and that guy at the party. You just didn't get caught.

ANTHONY: My God, that's not the same thing. Everybody does that sometimes. But that's not the point. The point is we agreed we wouldn't have full-fledged sex with anybody else. For love and safety of each other. You broke your word. Again! Just admit it.

KEVIN: Yes. I broke my word. I did. But about that, not about anything else between us. But you could've broken your word too and just didn't get infected.

This was such a loaded issue that it took several attempts to break in and interrupt their cycle to assess further. It was important to de-escalate their mutual accusation pattern and have them articulate their emotional experiences of this break in trust. Once they had a better understanding of each partner's respective experiences and needs, they might (but not always) be better equipped to restructure their interactions more successfully.

THERAPIST: Let's try and understand what happened for both of you. Can either of you start us off?

KEVIN: He's always accusing me of betraying him. I mean always and I don't know what else to say. I feel like you hate me and yet you want me to keep coming for more punishment. . . .

ANTHONY: Well you act like nothing much happened, and I feel like you're ready to just move on . . . as if nothing happened, in terms of you betraying me. How could I be anything other than hurt and suspicious now?

KEVIN: [Snidely] Tell me what to do and I'll do it. You want me to call you everywhere I go, every time I'm a couple of minutes late. Is that what you want?

What emerged was a dynamic in which Kevin pursued Anthony, Anthony became distant to protect himself, and the more he did, the more anxious Kevin became. The pattern was established and maintained with each inducing further insecurity in the other. Similar to the way they related regarding fear of HIV transmission in their relationship, they formulated a pattern that maintained their distance about Anthony's sense of betrayal because they were both fearful of rejection.

The attachment injury that Johnson, Makinen, and Millikin (2001) discussed was evident between Kevin and Anthony. Always ambivalent about becoming dependent on Anthony, Kevin tried to maintain a level of individuation that threatened the survival of their attachment. Anthony, who had felt insecure from the beginning of the relationship when Kevin was conflicted about moving in and agreeing and committing to monogamy, now felt betrayed and mistrustful. The HIV diagnosis, was, as Anthony says, "the evidence" of Kevin's betrayal, and now Anthony feels he can never trust or depend on Kevin again.

Given the gravity of this injury, work went slowly and deeply, trying to help these partners to reestablish even limited trust. As different issues emerged, and empathic alliances were renewed around other conflicts, the issue of trust and betrayal continued to reemerge. By using dyadic facilitation and interpretation, Kevin and Anthony were helped to understand how each of their preexisting trust issues early in life had laid the blueprint for some of the emotional reactions they experienced with each other.

Kevin's primary caregiver was a reluctant mother who often tried to do the right things, but appeared to "have her heart and mind elsewhere" as reported by Kevin. With peers, he felt like a "phony," and was afraid to be found out and fearful of being rejected if they suspected he might be gay. On coming out as a young adult he experienced rejection and abandonment by key figures. His attachment style seemed to be both ambivalent and insecure.

Anthony's attachment history was similar. He recalls primary relationships as evaluative. He often felt judged and appreciated only very conditionally. If he did shine at home, it was a threat to his father and he was duly punished by emotional withdrawal from his dad. In peer relationships and early romantic relationships, he often played "second fiddle" to keep his boyfriend happy and often chose partners that were untrustworthy and needed him to be their sidekick. Anthony struggled to confront Kevin because he was afraid of Kevin's disapproval and/or emotional withdrawal. Anthony's feelings of betrayal colored all of their conflicts and all of their interactions, and until he was able to gain insight (from individual therapy) about his need to replicate his early feelings of rejection and even betrayal, the overall prognosis for this couple repairing and establishing trust again was guarded.

SUMMARY

Although feelings of mistrust and betrayal are not typically found among serodiscordant couples, it is a dynamic that was identified as a strong concern for approximately 20 percent. Learning of one's partner's positive HIV status at any stage of the relationship may create some feelings of mistrust or even betrayal. One common scenario takes place when a couple assumes they share an HIV negative status, and then an HIV positive is revealed. This may very well threaten the growing trust of an early relationship. The second scenario involves a couple who has been HIV negative, with an established understanding of monogamy or safer sex outside of the relationship, and then becomes serodiscordant as a result of an unsafe sex episode of one partner outside of the relationship. Whenever and however this break in trust occurs between partners, it provokes profound feelings of hurt and betrayal. With such high emotional reactivity, early stages of couple therapy might do better with more behaviorally oriented approaches, such as structural or crisis, rather than emotionally oriented approaches.

Chapter 11

HIV and Family Planning

OVERVIEW

Although issues surrounding family planning and HIV were not identified as a primary concern for the majority of couples of mixed HIV status in this study, 28 percent of respondents (n = 25) agreed it was of some concern in their relationship. As the face of HIV/AIDS has become more feminine over the past decade, there has been an increase in implications for family planning in couples (Beckerman, Beder, and Gelman, 1996; Cates and Stone, 1992). Regardless of which partner was HIV positive, couples live with fears of passing HIV infection to their unborn children, as well as the fear that one partner would be too ill to parent. Even with techniques to reduce HIV by sperm washing and the use of triple combination therapy with pregnant HIV-positive women (which can greatly reduce the risk of passing HIV to unborn children), HIV was seen as an unyielding obstacle to starting a family (Beckerman, Beder, and Gelman, 1996; Gilman and Newman, 1996; CDC, 1994; Hutchinson and Kurth, 1991; Sonnenberg-Schwa et al., 1993).

QUANTITATIVE FINDINGS

Of the six issues that emerged as common to couples of mixed HIV status, family planning demonstrated the largest variation according to sexual orientation (Table 11.1). Thirty percent of heterosexual couples strongly agreed that family planning was a primary concern in their relationship. Several gay male couples identified conflict regarding their wish to become parents as it has been affected by an

TABLE 11.1. Sexual orientation: Family planning issues are of primary concern.

	Strongly agree	Agree	Disagree	Strongly disagree	Total
Heterosexual	12 (30%)	10 (25%)	11 (27.5%)	7 (17.5%)	40
Homosexual	0	3 (6%)	28 (58%)	17 (35%)	48
Total	12	13	39	24	88

HIV diagnosis, but only 6 percent of gay male couples identified family planning per se as a primary concern.

When exploring how family planning issues affect couples of mixed HIV status, gender is a paramount variable. For women, HIV may represent the loss regarding motherhood. A central concern for women is the worry and guilt that if they were HIV positive they might transmit HIV to their unborn child (Beckerman, 2000). For many women of childbearing age in serodiscordant relationships, HIV "shattered their dream, hopes and expectations" that they would become mothers (Beckerman, 2000, p. 13). HIV has signaled the loss of their role as a mother, which has been arguably more central to women's identities than the role of a father to men in mainstream society.

In this study, 50 percent of the women (n = 10) strongly agreed, and when collapsing the two categories of agreement, nearly the entire female sample identified family planning as a primary concern in their serodiscordant relationship (Table 11.2). Family planning was experienced as a primary concern for 3 percent of men. In fact, 91 percent disagreed that family planning was of concern. Of course, half of the males in the study are in gay male relationships, which may explain the overwhelming disagreement with this issue.

Within heterosexual serodiscordant relationships, family planning issues were of course highest for women who had tested HIV positive, then HIV-negative women, and of relatively little importance to men regardless of their serostatus (Table 11.3). This is a very small sample of heterosexual serodiscordant partners, but it does confirm

TABLE 11.2. Gender in heterosexual relationships: Family planning issues are of primary concern.

	Strongly agree	Agree	Disagree	Strongly disagree	Total
Female	10 (50%)	9 (45%)	1 (5%)	0	20
Male	2 (3%)	4 (6%)	38 (56%)	24 (35%)	68
Total	12	13	39	24	88

TABLE 11.3. HIV-positive partners in heterosexual relationships: Family planning issues are of primary concern.

	Strongly agree	Agree	Disagree	Strongly disagree	Total
HIV-positive women	7 (70%)	3 (30%)	0	0	10
HIV-positive men	0	0	4 (40%)	6 (60%)	10
HIV-negative women	3 (30%)	6 (60%)	1 (10%)	0	10
HIV-negative men	0	1 (10%)	5 (50%)	4 (40%)	10
Total	10	10	10	10	40

other research, empirical and anecdotal, that suggests women experience a great deal more stress regarding the impact on family planning than their male partners do (Walker, 1991).

Throughout the study, there was little or no difference between representatives of different ethnicities (Table 11.4). However, when it came to how family planning impacted the life of a couple of mixed HIV status, variations among ethnicities was evident. Family planning concerns were more commonly reported by African-American and Hispanic couples than white couples. More than a half of African-American couples and more than a third of Hispanic couples identified family planning issues as a primary concern, while approximately 10 percent of white couples identified it as such. A disproportionate number of younger women, socioeconomically disadvantaged women, and women of color are infected with HIV (Tangenberg, 2003). Relevant HIV literature would explain that among ethnicities and cultures, the role of motherhood continues to be a primary, if not sole, source of value (Tangenberg, 2003).

One's serostatus was not a significant indicator of their level of concern regarding family planning in their relationship (Table 11.5). There was, however, a somewhat higher response from those partners who were HIV positive (38 percent when agree categories are col-

TABLE 11.4. Ethnicity: Family planning issues are of primary concern.

	Strongly agree	Agree	Disagree	Strongly disagree	Total
African American	7 (30%)	6 (26%)	8 (35%)	2 (9%)	23
Hispanic	3 (11%)	6 (21%)	16 (57%)	3 (11%)	28
White	2 (5%)	1 (3%)	15 (41%)	19 (51%)	37
Total	12	13	39	24	88

TABLE 11.5. Serostatus: Family planning issues are of primary concern.

	Strongly agree	Agree	Disagree	Strongly disagree	Total
HIV positive	8 (18%)	9 (20%)	21 (48%)	6 (14%)	44
HIV negative	4 (9%)	4 (9%)	18 (41%)	18 (41%)	44
Total	12	13	39	24	88

lapsed) than their HIV-negative partners (18 percent) when it came to identifying concern about family planning issues. This difference most likely represents the intensity with which HIV-positive partners fear passing the virus onto their unborn child in ways more profound than their partners can identify.

The length of a relationship was not a major factor as to whether a couple experienced family planning issues (Table 11.6). However, unlike previous issues that presented more concern for newer couples, family planning issues appeared to arise in longer-term relationships.

When faced with emotional challenges, a consistent predictor of the level of concern has been when the couple learned of their serodiscordance. Couples who learned of the diagnosis early in their courtship consistently fared better than those who were diagnosed later in their relationship. The one departure in this pattern emerges when serodiscordant couples face family planning issues. More than 18 percent of couples who were diagnosed before their relationship identified family planning as a primary concern and 34 percent of couples who learned of their HIV diagnosis after their relationship was established identified concern regarding HIV and family planning. A possible inference may be drawn that family planning conversations between partners may not have occurred early in courtship as it might in an established relationship. One can also see the contradiction that a larger majority (81.5 percent) of those diagnosed before the relationship disagreed that this was an issue, whereas 66 percent of those who learned of their serodiscordance in their relationship disagreed as seen in Table 11.7.

TABLE 11.6. Length of relationship: Family planning issues are of primary concern.

	Strongly agree	Agree	Disagree	Strongly disagree	Total
Less than 5 years	4 (11%)	5 (13%)	21 (55%)	8 (21%)	38
More than 5 years	8 (16%)	8 (16%)	18 (36%)	16 (32%)	50
Total	12	13	39	24	88

When it comes to family planning concerns, there is a stark difference between those who have and have not experienced HIV-related illness (Table 11.8). Combining strongly agree and agree, only 14 percent of those who have experienced an HIV-related illness reported that family planning issues were of primary concern. Compare this with those couples who had not experienced an HIV-related illness, 50 percent of whom experienced concern regarding family planning with their partner. In the light (or the dark) of illness, wishes about the future often recede as the concern of illness predominates. It may be that while a partner is asymptomatic, the couple has a level of optimism about their future that can be temporarily interrupted by illness. Once the couple has experienced the crisis of medical illness, HIV may present a different level of reality that feels inconsistent with family planning.

TABLE 11.7. When couple learned of HIV diagnosis: Family planning issues are of primary concern.

	Strongly agree	Agree	Disagree	Strongly disagree	Total
Diagnosed before relationship	2 (6%)	4 (12.5%)	6 (19%)	20 (62.5%)	32
Diagnosed in relationship	10 (18%)	9 (16%)	33 (59%)	4 (7%)	56
Total	12	13	39	24	88

TABLE 11.8. HIV-related illness: Family planning issues are of primary concern.

	Strongly agree	Agree	Disagree	Strongly disagree	Total
Have had HIV illness	1 (2%)	6 (12%)	21 (40%)	24 (46%)	52
Have not had HIV illness	11 (31%)	7 (19%)	18 (50%)	0	36
Total	12	13	39	24	88

QUALITATIVE FINDINGS

Narrative Responses

When asked whether their difference in HIV status affected their feelings about becoming parents and creating a family, respondents consistently described HIV as interrupting their natural wishes and abilities to create a family. Two different scenarios emerged in their responses. The first, which affects only heterosexual serodiscordant couples, is the fear of infecting an unborn child, either by an HIV-positive woman passing HIV onto her unborn child or an HIV-positive male fearing he may pass HIV onto his female partner and unborn child.

The second scenario involves heterosexual and gay male couples and revolves around the fear of disease progression in one parent rendering him or her unable to share in child-rearing responsibilities. Should the HIV-positive partner become seriously ill, not only would he or she be unable to care for the child, he or she may require intensive caretaking. It seems these fears were experienced by several male couples who were exploring the idea of becoming parents through surrogacy or adoption and then retreated for fear that as a couple of mixed HIV status, they would not have the luxury to plan having a child as if HIV was not going to progress. Responses about family planning issues and how they were experienced is provided here.

Fear of Transmitting Virus to Partner/Unborn Child

> "He is not willing to make a baby with me. I wish we could have kids the old-fashioned way, but I know he's right."

> "I want to have more children so bad, but I know I could pass this on. It's one of the saddest things that my boyfriend and I won't have kids together."

> "I just never thought I'd feel so strong about this, but I feel like my life is over because we can't have kids together."

> "I want to become a mother, but I'm positive and I just can't take the chance of harming my baby."

Fear That HIV-Positive Partner Will Be Unable to Share Parenting and May Require Caretaking

> "What if we had a baby and then the baby was healthy, but I got sicker. I wouldn't be able to take care of the baby."

> "I just don't know how long we have that I'm still in good health. Not only wouldn't I be there to help with a kid, I may need her to take care of me. A kid is just out of the question."

> "We talk about adopting and fight. I really want to have kids and to be a parent. My health is fine. I feel I can handle it, but he just won't consider it because he feels it's not fair to the kid or me if he gets sick."

Case Studies

Case I: Hank and Lil

Hank is a forty-one-year-old man who is currently married to his second wife, Lil. Hank has had several ongoing relationships with men, but does not identify himself as gay and has not been "out" to his friends, family, or wife. He is a successful architect in private practice. He comes from a chaotic family in which both parents were alcoholics, and his brother has been clinically depressed, underachieving, and socially isolated for most of his life. Hank has been "the normal one" in the family, completing college, marrying young, and having a daughter. Unfortunately, he felt estranged from his wife and child and suffered panic attacks through much of his first marriage. He had several affairs with men, and several years into his first marriage he began an affair with a male acquaintance that ended abruptly when his boyfriend forced him to make a decision between him and staying married. Hank chose to stay married, but shortly after his breakup with his boyfriend, his wife asked for a divorce due to her dissatisfaction with their marriage.

He met his current wife, Lil through mutual friends. They dated for several years before they got married three years ago. While they were dating, Hank and Lil got tested. He tested positive and she tested negative. Lil is a thirty-five-year-old musician who also works as a house painter. Hank assumed that, for many reasons, he and Lil would not consider having children, HIV being the most significant reason. Lil wants very much to have children with Hank, and Hank feels this is out of the question, and will not consider sperm-washing or adoption. His health is stable and his viral load is consistently low, which has left him in an emotional limbo, waiting for illness to appear. Lil feels his good health may not always continue and feels an urgency to live fully by having children. These emotional responses to good health due to combination therapies has been coined the "protease moment," in which all is tentatively well, and for some partners, time stops while they wait for the illness to appear, and for others, they have an urgency to live as fully as possible (Greenan and Tunnell, 2003).

Hank and Lil have been fighting over the past year about a variety of issues, including money, sex, and having children. Hank presented as depressed and anxious to reduce the conflict between them. Lil presented as wanting to win the several power struggles they are entangled in and move them out of their rut. Several excerpts regarding family planning issues between this couple are provided to demonstrate how this issue might present itself and how emotionally focused couple therapy may facilitate a more adaptive conflict resolution.

HANK: She's just become very insistent, and so when we talk about anything, she's can't look at how she comes off. She doesn't really know she's become very aggressive. If I don't fight back, she'll walk all over me.

THERAPIST: So your perception is that she has become more certain about what she wants and has been pushing more toward it, and you feel it has become necessary to stick to your guns in the face of her pressure?

HANK: Yes. I feel, if she could back up a bit and be reasonable, I could be more flexible. There are just some things we can do and some things we're not going to be able to do. No matter how much she pushes.

LIL: What would you have me do? Give up on everything because you don't want to do it. Should I stop living because you have. No movies, no interest in going out, no sex, don't spend money, don't have kids. What is it you want to do? Just sit on the couch and wait to get sick?

HANK: Can you hear how you come off? Can you hear how shrill you are? You're not being reasonable. Like now's the time to have kids? I wish you could hear yourself.

THERAPIST: Okay. Let's see if we can find a new way of working on this together. I can hear both of you. I hear that you are both very frustrated with one another, that you feel your partner is being unreasonable and stubborn and blaming. Is that in the right ballpark? [Hank and Lil both nod, and seem somewhat less angry.]

THERAPIST: There's sort of a sense that both of you feel you have to fight to get your point across or the other one will barrel over you? [They both nod.] So you are actually feeling some of the same things even though you think your partner doesn't understand how you feel?

With this realization, the mood in the room has softened significantly and the initial steps of EFCT are applied: de-escalating the cycle of maladaptive patterns and showing how these patterns have sustained negative feelings for each partner. Hank and Lil were each asked to focus more on their own emotional experiences than how they perceived each other. With this, the emphasis shifts from mutual accusation to empathic joining of presenting their emotional experiences.

THERAPIST: Lil, what have you been feeling about having kids with Hank?

LIL: To me, that's the next step. It's a step that brings us closer again and into building a future. I think it's the most important thing because I feel it is a way of going toward the future and not staying stuck. I know we would be great parents and I know he would be happier.

THERAPIST: So in some ways, for you Lil, having kids moves the two of you out of a rut and moves you toward a fuller future together? And you're very much thinking of him . . . that having kids would make him happier? Trying to help him out of what you see as a rut?

LIL: Yes. I mean I want to have kids and I know he does also. I don't think we shouldn't because of his health. I feel the opposite. His health is good and if we keep our spirits optimistic, he will do and feel better. I don't want to just give up the way he has. I don't want to let him give up.

THERAPIST: Hank, what did you hear about Lil's feelings about having kids?

HANK: Well. It did sound different this time around. I don't know. It sounded like she's doing it for me almost. But I really don't think that's the case. She's wants to have kids and it would be great if I did too. But I think this is for her, for her future and her spirits. The next big project she can throw herself into.

LIL: What if it's for both of us? Can't you even begin to consider that we can still make a good life? I feel like you've given up. I just don't understand why we can't even consider it.

HANK: I feel like you just can't accept that I don't want to have kids. I might have been talked into it before the HIV, but I can't anymore. I can't understand why you would keep pushing this.

At this juncture, both partners were more able to express their feelings about family planning without accusation, but still remained at a standstill. The aim was not necessarily to resolve their conflicting wishes, but to enable them to understand and empathize with their respective needs. In this way the harsh positioning that resulted in destructive encounters would be diffused. Middle stages focused on building empathy with each other and helping to explore some of their underlying emotional issues that fueled their interactional positioning.

THERAPIST: Hank, can you help Lil understand why you feel kids are out of the picture for you?

HANK: I feel like she doesn't accept that in some areas, I did give up. It just doesn't make sense for us to have kids. [Long pause, then he confronts Lil.] What if I get sick? How are you going to take care of a child and me?

THERAPIST: Can you explain to Lil what you worry about, when you think of that?

HANK: I just think it's crazy. What if we have a baby, the baby can be perfectly healthy, but what if I get sick? What if she's alone taking care of the baby and then what if she has to take care of me also?

LIL: I would do whatever I have to. [She starts crying.] Is that what this is about? You're afraid I won't be able to take care of you?

HANK: It's not what it's about. It's one thing. I worry about a million things. That's just one thing I'd worry about.

THERAPIST: I'm sure both of you worry about different things in different ways. Those worries make you take the stand you've taken. Lil, even if you see things differently, are you able to let Hank know that you understand these worries he has about how kids would make things different?

LIL: I don't know. It seems like such a shame. Such a loss.

THERAPIST: Can you let him know that you're trying to understand how he feels . . . and maybe explain what sort of things you worry about in terms of this issue?

LIL: [Long pause and then directly to Hank] I am trying. I just don't worry that way. I worry more that we're just waiting for you to get sick. What's the point of taking your meds and being healthy if we've stopped living.

As Hank and Lil expanded on their worries about having kids, the session moved further into their unacknowledged feelings and some of the attachment issues and conflicts that were being provoked by this family planning struggle. Over the next several sessions, therapy emphasized insight-oriented interventions and interpretations that helped them explore and identify how early attachment conflicts and patterns were being repeated in this conflict with each other.

Hank was able to identify and understand that in his emotionally and functionally chaotic family of origin, he survived by being emotionally independent. As his needs for attachment and security often went unmet, he developed an insecure attachment style marked by separation anxiety, panic attacks, and a looming sense that each attachment would become unpredictable and insecure. Over the next several sessions, Hank and Lil learned together how the idea of having children was intolerable to him on numerous levels. At the crux of his disdain for the idea was that it symbolized a loss of Lil. He articulated that he felt he would lose her to the baby and this was something he could not risk, particularly now because he feared he would need her full attention and support if he became ill. He was able to own this need and express it in a way that Lil could join with him and understand and even begin to let go of her need.

Lil was able to understand her need to have a child with Hank on a deeper level as well. Her tenacity with this issue belied her anxiety "to beat" the HIV and, in some ways, keep Hank involved in life-affirming activities. Intensive work was done with both Hank and Lil and there were moments for Lil that brought clarity to her need for having children now. These were needs that can also be understood through the attachment lens—needs for security and stability. The need for humans to attach and build secure attachments, a safe haven, is universal (Bowlby, 1969). Interestingly, this emerged with clarity when Hank asked Lil what having kids together would do for her (not him).

LIL: [Weary and defeated] I'm just tired of worrying and waiting. I feel like I've been doing that my whole life about one thing or another and I'm just ready to settle down and be in the moment. Not worry about the future, but build something stable. It's about my music, it's about my history. I just want to build something that's just ours, that's safe and sturdy. I just want to be a family. I want to have a family.

HANK: [After silence in the room] I'm sorry I can't give you that. Not the way you want it.

With the expression of needs and wants and an empathic emotional engagement, there can be conflict resolution that is mutually satisfactory to both partners. In this scenario, Hank and Lil felt much closer, but the conflict resolution was one that relieved and saddened Hank and left Lil feeling defeated. Sometimes, even with a couple that is highly motivated and capable and has insight and empathy, a perfect outcome is still unattainable. Later stages of EFCT resulted in the facilitation of a safe and constructive avenue for each partner to be forthcoming about their emotional experiences. This foundation provides them with more adaptive emotional patterns and more constructive interactional positioning with each other. With more empathetically attuned positions, Hank and Lil may avoid destructive injuries and disengagement, and may even be able to resolve other issues in a mutually satisfactory way.

Case II: Mike and Claude

Mike and Claude, a serodiscordant couple who were seen for nearly a year, faced issues regarding fear of HIV transmission and disclosure that were discussed in Chapters 6 and 9. They had planned to adopt children until they found out that Mike was HIV positive. With his diagnosis, they both became conflicted about pursuing parenthood. Each is ambivalent about this issue and they provoke each other to externalize their internalized conflict. A combination of structural and emotionally focused couple therapy was used to help them address their conflict more constructively.

Key concepts from structural therapy such as roles, homeostasis, and hierarchy were explored and reframed. As a result of therapy, Mike and Claude had entered consciously into emotional roles that were increasingly adaptive and flexible. In many ways, they had successfully negotiated their conflicts around HIV transmission and disclosure. The crisis surrounding the issue of family planning had yet to be addressed.

As Claude tried to pursue talking about adopting a child, Mike often responded by being dismissive and then withdrawing. This heightened Claude's sense of rejection and loss, as they had been joined in their excitement about becoming parents. Mike would respond to Claude's withdrawal by apologizing for being HIV positive, and Claude often felt he was not supposed to be angry or disappointed about not becoming parents because it would just upset Mike further.

This opened up the area of how power is organized and how HIV had changed the unspoken norms of who held which forms of power in this relationship. Since the diagnosis, Claude has felt that his role was to be supportive and protective to Mike. Increasingly, he avoided expressing disagreement because he did not want to cause Mike further stress. In a way, Mike became more powerful with the diagnosis, and Claude felt "smaller and smaller" and that he should "bow to Mike's needs and wishes." Once this shift was identified, Mike and Claude shared a wish to return to the way they operated before. Mike did not wish to "be babied or treated with kid gloves," that in fact such treatment made him feel more depressed. From this discussion, a new contract emerged that Mike and Claude would be fully honest even if this caused disagreement or stress for Mike.

Emotionally focused therapy was also applied to help Mike and Claude "soften" their positions about family planning,

CLAUDE: I just feel angry and frustrated about not having kids. I just can't believe it.

MIKE: I can't help it. Don't you think I wish this didn't happen? What do you want me to do?

THERAPIST: Before we go further, I see that the way you're bringing up your feelings, Claude, causes Mike to feel he has to defend himself. In addition to feeling angry and frustrated, what are some of your other feelings that may not put him on the defensive.

CLAUDE: I feel sad. I feel really disappointed. I can't have kids without him. I don't want kids without him. I think we should still consider having kids.

THERAPIST: [Facilitating empathic joining] Even if your wishes are different, where is there some overlap between how you both feel?

MIKE: I know he's going through a lot of what I am going through. I know in terms of having kids, he's frustrated and totally let down.

CLAUDE: In that way, we're both bummed out, most of the time. The kids are one thing, but you know we're frustrated by so many things about our sex life, who to tell, what to plan for. . . . It's all been blown to shit. And I guess the kid thing feels like the last straw to me. It's like, can't we get anything we wanted?

With this, there was a palpable shift in the room from anger and frustration to sadness. The feelings of grief and loss were expressed, and both partners were able to sustain the discomfort of their individual and shared sadness. Mike and Claude became visibly closer, moving next to each other and holding hands as they talked about what they felt they lost the day the diagnosis came back positive. There was a sad resolution in that session that Mike and Claude would not pursue becoming parents. Claude felt he heard for the first time that Mike was just incapable, and that while Mike may "flip-flop" and sometimes talk about having kids, they both knew that "that was just talk" because it was difficult for Mike to give up becoming a parent as well. With realignment of roles, softening of their communication patterns, and attention to shoring up their emotional engagement with each other, Mike and Claude were helped to come to several viable resolutions about their life after the HIV diagnosis. Most important, they left therapy feeling significantly closer and more capable of negotiating their conflicts without adding further injury to the relationship.

SUMMARY

Heterosexual couples overwhelmingly expressed the intense conflict over whether to have children given the presence of HIV in their life. Homosexual couples also identified this as an emotional challenge in open-ended responses. Practitioners should anticipate the likelihood that serodiscordant couples are contending with the emotional challenges related to desires to be pregnant and raise children. Alternatives such as semen washing are now available among reproductive specialists, and information and referral should be provided as possible alternatives where the male is HIV infected.

The therapist can assist the couple to clarify how HIV-related fears, anxieties, and disappointments may be affecting the emotional life of each partner individually and as a couple. Here, as with other emotional challenges, there exists a delicate balance between mourning the loss of not having children and assisting the couple in their life-affirming adaptations.

Epilogue

Every couple who is faced with a medical crisis of one partner will experience a range of intrapsychic emotional responses and relationship challenges. When seeking assistance with adaptation to illness or potential illness in their lives, as in asymptomatic HIV, couples will pose a variety of challenges to a couple therapist. The shifting realities of HIV/AIDS, the sociocultural and characterological factors, family histories, and historical and current injuries in the relationship will all present themselves in different ways for each couple and with each different therapist. Numerous couple frameworks might be differentially applied to both universal and unique dyadic challenges facing couples of mixed HIV status.

Emotionally focused couple therapy, with an emphasis on the rejuvenation of empathic bonds between partners and the uncovering of underlying attachment issues, can effectively guide a therapist in assessment and intervention with couples coping with HIV. Integrative couple therapy can guide a therapist in ways emotionally focused therapy does not emphasize, identifying those behaviors that need to be shifted and accepting those behaviors that can be shifted by respective partners. Medical family therapy, largely based on crisis with some concepts from the structural approach as well, can be used to facilitate more adaptive coping to the emotional impact of illness in a couple's life. Each of these approaches and others can be applied to the unique dyadic challenges facing couples of mixed HIV status, but this book asserts that a particularly relevant theoretical framework is emotionally focused couple therapy. Universal and unique emotional issues of attachment and attachment injury lend themselves to the texture of the types of issues that commonly face couples of mixed HIV status, such as fear of HIV transmission, shifts in emotional intimacy, coping with the uncertainty attendant to HIV, disclosure issues, mistrust/betrayal, and family planning. Many conflictual issues can be conceptualized as stemming from underlying attachment issues; issues that are triggered by the presence of a potentially life-threaten-

ing illness. In understanding some of the common emotional challenges HIV may raise, considering the application of EFCT and other
approaches, the therapist may be better equipped to diminish some of
the struggle between partners at a time when they need each other the
most.

References

Adam, B. and Sears, A. (1994). Negotiating sexual relationships after testing HIV positive. *Medical Anthropology 16* (1), 63-77.

Adam, B.D. and Sears, A. (1996). *Experiencing HIV: Personal, Family, and Work Relationships.* New York: Columbia University Press.

Alexander, J.F., Holtzworth-Munroe, A., and Jameson, P. (1994). The process and outcome of marital and family therapy: Research review and evaluation. In A. Bergin and S. Garfield (Eds.), *Handbook of Psychotherapy and Behavior Change* (pp. 595-607). New York: Wiley.

Anderson, W. and Weatherburn, P. (1998). *The Impact of Combination Therapy on the Illness of People with HIV.* London: Sigma Research.

Avert, D. (2002). HIV and pregnancy: Tough choices . . . and the right to choose. *The Journal of the Association of Nurses in AIDS Care 13*(3), 11-12.

Bacon, L. (1987). Lessons of AIDS: Racism, and homophobia are the real epidemic. *Listen Real Loud 8*(2), 5-7.

Baider, L. and Sarell, M. (1984). Couples in crisis: Patient-spouse differences in perception of interactive patterns and the illness situation. *Family Therapy, 11*(2), 112-122.

Baider, R. and Spexiele, B.A. (1997) Couples' sexual intimacy and multiple sclerosis. *Journal of Family Psychotherapy 8*(1), 13-22.

Barrett, R.L. (1989). Counseling gay men with AIDS: The human dimensions. *Journal of Counseling and Development 67*(4), 573-575.

Baucom, D.H. and Epstein, N. (1990). *Cognitive-Behavioral Marital Therapy.* New York: Brunner/Mazel.

Baucom, D.H. and Hoffman, J.A. (1986). The effectiveness of marital therapy: Current status and application to the clinical setting. In N. Jacobsen and A. Gurman (Eds.), *Clinical Handbook of Marital Therapy* (pp. 597-620). New York: The Guilford Press.

Baucom, D.H., Sayers, S.L., and Sheer, T.G. (1990). Supplementing behavioral marital therapy with cognitive restructuring and emotional expressiveness training: An outcome investigation. *Journal of Consulting and Clinical Psychology 58,* 636-645.

Baucom, D.H., Shoham, V., Mueser, K., Daiuto, A., and Stickle, T. (1998). Empirically supported couple and family interventions for marital distress and adult mental health problems. *Journal of Consulting and Clinical Psychology 66,* 53-88.

Beckerman, N.L. (2000). The impact of HIV on women's relationships: Implications for the direct practitioner. *Practice 12*(1), 5-16.

Beckerman, N.L. and Auerbach, C. (2002). Couples of mixed HIV status: Psychosocial issues affecting intimacy. *Journal of Couple and Relationship Therapy 1*(4), 73-85.

Beckerman, N.L., Beder, J., and Gelman, S.R. (1996). Mandatory HIV testing of newborns: The debate and a programmatic response. *Affilia 11*(4), 462-483.

Beckerman, N.L. and Gelman, S.R. (2000). A shift in HIV reporting practices: A biopolitical analysis. *Journal of Health and Social Policy 12*(2), 73-87.

Beckerman, N.L. and Grube, B. (2003). Hepatitis C and HIV: What social workers need to know. *Journal of Case Management 3*(4), 114-118.

Beckerman, N.L., Letteney, S., and Lorber, K. (2001). Emotional issues of serodiscordant couples. *Social Work in Health Care 31*(4), 25-41.

Bor, R., Miller, R., and Goldman, E. (1993). *Theory and Practice of HIV Counseling: A Systemic Approach.* New York: Brunner/Mazel.

Bowen, M. (1978). *Family Therapy in Clinical Practice.* New York: James Aronson.

Bowlby, J. (1969). *Attachment and Loss,* Volume 1: *Attachment.* New York: Basic Books.

Bowlby, J. (1988). *A Secure Base.* New York: Basic Books.

Buckingham, S.L. (1987). The HIV antibody test: Psychosocial issues. *Social Casework 68,* 387-393.

Burgoyne, W. (1994). Counseling gay male couples living with HIV. *Canadian Journal of Human Sexuality 3*(1), 1-14.

Cadwell, S. (1991). Twice removed: The stigma suffered by gay men with AIDS. *Smith College Studies in Social Work 61,* 236-246.

Campbell, T. and Patterson, J. (1995). The effectiveness of family interventions in the treatment of physical illness. *Journal of Marital and Family Therapy 21*(4), 543-583.

Carruthers, S.J., Loxley, W.M., Phillips, M., and Bevan, S. (2001). The study of HIV injecting drug use predicting exposure to Hepatitis C. *Drug and Alcohol Review 16*(3), 215-220.

Cates, W. and Stone, K.M. (1992). Family planning, sexually transmitted diseases, and contraceptive choices: A literature update. *Family Planning Perspectives 24,* 75-84.

Centers for Disease Control (CDC) (1981). Pneumocystis pneumonia-Los Angeles. *Morbidity and Mortality Weekly Reports 30,* 250-252.

Centers for Disease Control and Prevention (CDC) (1994). Zidovudine for the prevention of HIV transmission from mother to infant. *Morbidity and Mortality Weekly Report 43,* 285-287.

Centers for Disease Control and Prevention (1999). HIV/AIDS surveillance report. *HIV/AIDS Surveillance Report 10*(2), 7.

Centers for Disease Control and Prevention (2000). HIV/AIDS surveillance report. *HIV/AIDS Surveillance Report 11*(1), 4.

Centers for Disease Control and Prevention (2001). HIV/AIDS surveillance report. *HIV/AIDS Surveillance Report 12*(2), 11.

Chidwick, A. and Borrill, J. (1996). Dealing with a life-threatening diagnosis: The experience of people with the human immunodeficiency virus. *AIDS Care 8*, 271-284.

Christ, G. and Wiener, L. (1984). Psychosocial issues in AIDS. *Social Work in Health Care 13*(1), 6-14.

Curran, J.W. (1983). AIDS—Two years later. *New England Journal of Medicine 309*, 609-611.

Dattilio, F.M. (1993). Cognitive techniques with couples and families. *The Family Journal 1*(1), 51-56.

Dattilio, F.M. (1994). Families in crisis. In F.M. Dattilio and A. Freeman (Eds.), *Cognitive-Behavioral Strategies in Crisis Intervention* (pp. 278-301). New York: The Guilford Press.

Dattilio, F.M. and Bevilacqua, J. (2000). *Comparative Treatments for Relationship Dysfunction.* New York: Springer.

Denenberg, D. (1990). *Women, AIDS, and Activism.* Boston: South End Press.

Dietrich, D. (2001). Studies on co-infection with HIV/HBV and HIV/HCV. Available online at <http://www.hivandhepatitis.com/hiv11060001.html>.

Doherty, W.J., Baird, M., and Becker, L. (1987). Family medicine and the biopsychosocial model: The road to integration. *Marriage and Family Review 10*, 51-70.

Dowdle, W.R. (1983). The epidemiology of AIDS. *Public Health Reports 98*, 308-312.

Dunn, R.L. and Schweibel, A. (1995). Meta-analytic review of marital therapy and outcome research. *Journal of Family Psychology 9*(1), 58-68.

Ellis, A. (1977). The nature of disturbed marital interactions. In A. Ellis and R. Geiger (Eds.), *Handbook of RET* (pp. 170-176). New York: The Guilford Press.

Ellis, A. and Harper, R.A. (1961). *A Guide to Rational Living.* Englewood Cliffs, NJ: Prentice-Hall.

Epstein, N. and Baucom, D.H. (1989). Cognitive-behavioral marital therapy. In A. Freeman, K.M. Simon, L.E. Butler, and H. Arkowitz (Eds.), *Comprehensive Book of Cognitive Therapy* (pp. 491-513). New York: Plenum Press.

Feeney, A.J. (1999). *Adult Romantic Attachment: Theory, Research, and Clinical Applications.* New York: The Guilford Press.

Foley, M., Skurnick, J.H., Kennedy, C.A., Valentin, R., and Louria, D.B. (1994). Family support for heterosexual partners in HIV serodiscordant couples. *AIDS 8* (10), 1483-1487.

Folkman, S., Chesney, M.A., and Christopher-Richards, A. (1994). Stress and coping in caregiving partners of men with AIDS. *Psychiatric Clinics of North America 17*, 35-53.

Frazier, P., Davis-Ali, S., and Dahl, K.E. (1995). Stressors, social support, and adjustment in kidney transplant patients and their spouses. *Social Work in Health Care 21*(2), 93-108.

Furstenburg, A.L. and Olsen, M.M. (1984). Social work and AIDS. *Social Work in Health Care 9*, 45-62.

Gers, S.B., Fuller, R.L., and Rush, J. (1986). Lovers of AIDS victims: Psychosocial stresses and counseling needs. *Death Studies 10*, 43-53.

Gilligan, C. (1982). *In a Different Voice: Psychological Theory and Women's Development*. Cambridge, MA: Harvard University Press.

Gilman, S. and Newman, B.S. (1996). Psychosocial concerns and strengths of women with HIV infection: An empirical study. *Families in Society: The Journal of Contemporary Human Services 77*(3), 131-141.

Gochros, H. (1992). The sexuality of gay men with HIV infection. *Social Work 37*(2), 105-108.

Goldstein, N. (1997). *The Gender Politics of HIV/AIDS in Women: Perspectives on the Pandemic in the United States*. New York: New York University Press.

Gotay, C.C. (1984). The experience of cancer during early and advanced stages: The view of patients and their mates. *Social Science and Medicine 18*, 605-613.

Gottman, J. (1999). *The Marriage Clinic: A Scientifically Based Marital Therapy*. New York: Norton.

Grace, W.C. (1994). HIV counseling research needs suggested by psychotherapy process and outcome studies. *Professional Psychology: Research and Practice 25*, 403-409.

Green, G. (1995). Sex, love, and seropositivity: Balancing the risks. In P. Aggleton, P. Davies, and G. Hart (Eds.), *AIDS: Safety, Sexuality and Risk* (pp. 144-158). London: Taylor Francis.

Greenan, D.E. and Tunnell, G. (2003). *Couple Therapy with Gay Men*. New York: The Guilford Press.

Greenberg, L.S. and Johnson, S.M. (1988). *Emotionally Focused Therapy for Couples*. New York: Guilford.

Grube, B., Beckerman, N.L., and Strug, D. (2003). Examining the unique stresses and rewards of HIV work: Then and now. *Journal of HIV/AIDS and Social Services 1*(2), 5-20.

Gurman, A.S, Kniskern, D.P., and Pinsof, W.M. (1986). Research on the process and outcome of marital and family therapy. In S. Garfield and A. Bergin (Eds.), *Handbook of Psychotherapy and Behavior Change*. New York: Wiley

Hahlweg, K. and Markman, H.J. (1988). Effectiveness of behavioral marital therapy: Empirical status of behavioral techniques in preventing and alleviating marital distress. *Journal of Consulting and Clinical Psychology 56*, 440-447.

Hahlweg, K., Schindler, and Brengelmann, D. (1984). Effects of behavioral marital therapy on couples: Communication and problem-solving skills. *Journal of Consulting and Clinical Psychology 52*(4), 553-566.

Hausman, K. (1983). AIDS panic brings lonely life to patients, gays. *Psychiatric News 3*, 19-20.

Hays, R.B., McKusick, L., Pollack, L., and Hilliard, R. (1993). Disclosing HIV seropositivity to significant others. *AIDS 7*, 425-431.

Hazan, C. and Shaver, P. (1987). Conceptualizing romantic love as an attachment process. *Journal of Personality and Social Psychology 52*, 511-524.

Hoffman, M.A. (1991). Counseling the HIV infected client: A psychosocial model for assessment and intervention. *Counseling Psychologist 19*, 467-542.

Hoffman, M.A. (1996). *Counseling Clients with HIV Disease*. New York: The Guilford Press.

Huggins, J., Elman, N., Baker, C., Forrester, R.G., and Lyter, D. (1991). Affective and behavioral responses of gay and bisexual men to HIV antibody testing. *Social Work 36*(1), 61-65.

Hutchinson, M. and Kurth, A. (1991). "I need to know that I have a choice . . .": A study of women, HIV, and reproductive decision-making. *AIDS Patient Care 5*(1), 17-25.

Jacobsen, N.S. (1991). Behavioral vs. insight-oriented marital therapy: Labels can be misleading. *Journal of Consulting and Clinical Psychology 61*(1), 85-93.

Jacobsen, N.S. and Addis, M.E. (1993). Research on couples and couple therapy: What do we know? Where are we going? *Journal of Consulting and Clinical Psychology 61*(85-93).

Jacobsen, N. and Christensen, A. (1996a). *Acceptance and Change in Couple Therapy*. New York: W.W. Norton and Co.

Jacobsen, N.S. and Christensen, A. (1996b). *Integrative Couples Therapy*. New York: Norton.

Johnson, S.M. (1988). Emotionally focused couple therapy. In F.M. Dattilio (Ed.), *Case Studies in Couple and Family Therapy* (pp. 450-472). New York: The Guilford Press.

Johnson, S.M. (1999). Straight to the heart, In J.M. Donovan (Ed.), *Short-Term Couple Therapy* (pp. 13-42). New York: The Guilford Press.

Johnson, S.M. and Greenberg, L.S. (1995). The emotionally focused approach to problems in adult attachment. In N.S. Jacobsen and A.S. Gurman (Eds.), *Clinical Handbook of Couple Therapy* (pp. 121-141). New York: The Guilford Press.

Johnson, S.M., Hunsley, J., Greenberg, L.S., and Schindler, D. (1999). The effects of emotionally focused marital therapy: A meta-analysis. *Clinical Psychology: Science and Practice 6*, 67-79.

Johnson, S.M., Makinen, J.A., and Millikin, J.W. (2001). Attachment injuries in couple relationships: A new perspective on impasses in couples therapy. *Journal of Marital and Family Therapy 27*, 145.

Johnson, S.M., and Williams-Keeler, L. (1998). Creating healing relationships for couples dealing with trauma: The use of emotionally focused couple therapy. *Journal of Marital and Family Therapy 24*, 25-40.

Josephson, S.B. (1997). *Correlates of HIV/AIDS disclosure*. Dissertation. Columbia University. New York: Columbia University Press.

Kaisch, K. and Anton-Culver, A. (1989). Psychological and social consequence of HIV exposure: Homosexuals in Southern California. *Psychology and Health 3*, 63-75.

Kalichman, S., and Nachimson, D. (1999). Self-efficacy and disclosure of HIV positive serostatus to sex partners. *Health Psychology 18*, 281-287.

Kaspar, B. (1989). Women and AIDS: A psychosocial perspective. *Affilia 4*, 7-22.

Katz, D.A. (1997). The profile of HIV infection in women: A challenge to the profession. *Social Work in Health Care 24*(3), 127-134.

Kennedy, C.A., Skurnick, J.H., Foley, M., and Louria, D.B. (1995). Gender differences in HIV-related psychological distress in heterosexual couples. *AIDS Care 7*(Suppl.), 33-38.

Klimes, I., Catalan, J., Garrod, A., Day, A., Bond, A., and Rizza, C. (1992). Partners of men with HIV infection and hemophilia: Controlled investigation of factors associated with psychological morbidity. *AIDS Care 4*, 149-156.

Klitzman, R. (1997). *Being Positive: The Lives of Men and Women with HIV*. New York: Ivan R. Dee, Inc.

Kramer, L. (1989). *Reports from the Holocaust: The Making of an AIDS Activist*. New York: St. Martin's Press.

Krausz, S. (1988). Illness and loss: Helping couples cope. *Clinical Social Work Journal 16*(1), 52-65.

Lambiase, L., Pozzi, G., Pravettoni, G., Caprioli, S. and Suter, F. (1994). The influence of HIV seropositivity on the emotional relationship between heterosexual couples. *International Conference on AIDS 10*(1):407.

Leask, C., Elford, J., Bor, R., Miller, R., and Johnson, M. (1997). Selective disclosure: A pilot investigation into changes in family relationships since HIV diagnosis. *Journal of Family Therapy 19*, 59-69.

Liberian, R.P. (1970). Behavioral approaches to couple and family therapy. *American Journal of Orthopsychiatry 40*, 106-118.

Lippmann, W.A., James, W.A., and Frierson, R.L. (1993). AIDS and the family: Implications for counseling. *AIDS Care 5*, 71-78.

Lyons, R. (1995). *Relationships in Chronic Illness and Disability*. Thousand Oaks, CA: Sage.

MacDonald, B. (1998). Issues in therapy with gay and lesbian clients. *Journal of Sex and Marital Therapy 24*, 165-190.

Mancilla, M. and Troshinsky, L. (2003). *Love in the Time of HIV: The Gay Man's Guide to Sex, Dating, and Relationships*. New York: The Guilford Press.

Marks, G., Bundek, N.I., Richardson, J.L., Ruiz, M.S., Maldonado, N., and Mason, H.R. (1992). Self-disclosure of HIV infection: Preliminary results from a sample of Hispanic men. *Health Psychology 11*, 300-306.

Martin, D. (1989). HIV infection and the gay community: Counseling and clinical issues. *Journal of Counseling and Development 68*, 67-72.

Martin, J. (1988). Psychological consequences of AIDS-related bereavement among gay men. *Journal of Consulting and Clinical Psychology 56*, 856-862.

Martin, J. and Dean, L. (1993). Effects of AIDS-related bereavement of HIV-related illness of psychological distress among gay men: A seven year longitudinal study. *Journal of Consulting and Clinical Psychology 61*, 94-103.

Mass, L. (1981). *Rare Cancer Seen in 41 Homosexuals. The New York Times,* July 3, p. A12, C4.

Mayer, R. and Wells, E. (1997). HIV negative women in serodiscordant couples. *HIV Frontline: A Newsletter for Professionals Who Counsel People Living with HIV 29,* 1-3.

McDaniel, S.H., Hepworth, J., and Doherty, N. (1995). *Medical Family Therapy.* New York: Wiley.

McKusick, L., Horstman, W., and Carfagni, A. (1983). Report on community reaction to AIDS. Paper presented at the Ninety-First Annual Convention of the *American Psychological Association,* December 4, 1983, Anaheim, California.

Merriam, S. (2002). *Qualitative Research in Practice: Discussion and Analysis.* San Francisco: Jossey-Bass.

Minuchin, S. (1984). *Families and Family Therapy.* Cambridge, MA: Harvard University Press.

Mohr, J.J. (1999). *Same-Sex Romantic Attachment: Theory, Research, and Clinical Applications.* New York: The Guilford Press.

Moore, J., Harrison, J.S., VanDevanter, N., Kennedy, C., Padian, N., Abrams, J., Lesondak, L.M., and O'Brien, T. (1998). Factors influencing relationship quality of serodiscordant heterosexual couples. In V.J. Derlega and A.P. Barbee (Eds.), *HIV and Social Integration.* Thousand Oaks, CA: Sage Publications.

Moore, J., VanDevanter, N., Padian, N., Skurnick, J., Jankowski, M., Bromberg, J., Cordell, J., and O'Brien, T.R. (1995). Women's safer sex communications with male partners: A study of HIV discordant couples. *HIV Infection Conference,* S56(1), 2-9.

Moos, R. and Tsu, V. (1977). The crisis of physical illness: An overview. In R. Moos and V. Tsu (Eds.), *Coping with Physical Illness.* New York: Plenum Press.

Neugenberger, R., Rabkin, J., Williams, J.B., Remien, R.H., Goetz, R., and Gorman, J. M. (1992). Bereavement reactions among homosexual men experiencing multiple losses in the AIDS epidemic. *American Journal of Psychiatry* 149, 1374-1379.

Padian, N.S., O'Brien, T.R., Chang, Y., Glass, S., and Francis, D.P. (1993). Prevention of heterosexual transmission of HIV through couple counseling. *Journal of Acquired Immunodefiency Syndrome 6,* 1043-1048.

Palmer, R. and Bor, R. (2001). The challenges to intimacy and sexual relationships for gay men in serodiscordant relationships: A pilot study. *Journal of Marital and Family Therapy 27*(4), 419-431.

Parad, H. (1965). *Crisis Intervention.* New York: Family Service Association.

Parker, G. (1993). Disability, caring, and marriage: The experiences of younger couples when a partner is disabled after marriage. *British Journal of Social Work 23*(6), 565-580.

Pasquier, C., Daudin, M., Righi, L., Berges, L., Thauvin, L., Berribi, A., Massip, P., Puel, J., Bujan, L., and Izopet, J. (2000). Sperm washing and virus nucleic acid detection to reduce HIV and hepatitis C virus transmission in serodiscordant couples wishing to have children. *AIDS 14,* 2093-2099.

Patterson, G.R. (1971). *Families: Applications of Social Learning to Family Life.* Champaign, IL: Research Press.

Pearlin, L.I., Semple, S., and Turner, G. (1993). Stress of AIDS caregiving: A preliminary overview of the issues. *Death Studies 12,* 501-547.

Poindexter, C.C. (2004). Unserved, unseen, and unheard: Integrating programs for HIV-infected and HIV-affected older adults. *Health and Social Work 29*(2), 86-95.

Pomeroy, E., Green, E., and Van Laningham, D. (2002). Couples who care: The effectiveness of a psychoeducational group intervention for HIV serodiscordant couples. *Research on Social Work Practice 12*(2), 238-252.

Powell-Cope, G.M. (1995). The experiences of gay couples affected by HIV infections. *Qualitative Health Research 5*(1), 36-62.

Powell-Cope, G.M. (1996). HIV disease symptom management in the context of committed relationships. *Journal of the Association of Nurses in AIDS Care 7*(3), 19-28.

Powell-Cope, G.M. and Brown, M.A. (1992). Going public as an AIDS family caregiver. *Social Science and Medicine 34,* 571-580.

Rait, D.S., Ross, J.M., and Rao, S.M. (1997). Treating couples and families with HIV: A systemic approach. In M.F. O'Connor, and I. Yalom (Eds.), *Treating the Psychological Consequences of HIV.* San Francisco: Jossey-Bass.

Remien, R. (1998). HIV medical advances and couples. *Focus: A Guide to AIDS Research and Counseling 13*(5), 1-4.

Remien, R., Carballo-Dieguez, A., and Wagner, G. (1995). Intimacy and sexual risk behavior in serodiscordant male couples. *AIDS Care 7,* 429-438.

Ripple, L. (1964). *Motivation, Capacity, and Opportunity in Casework Theory.* Chicago: Chicago University Press.

Rolland, J.S. (1994). In sickness and in health: The impact of illness on couples' relationships, *Journal of Marital and Family Therapy 20,* 327-347.

Rowe, W., Plum, G., and Crossman, C. (1988). Issues and problems confronting the lovers, families, and communities associated with persons with AIDS. *Journal of Social Work and Human Sexuality 6*(2),110-124.

Sabo, D., Brown, J., and Smith, C. (1986). The male role and mastectomy: Support groups and men's adjustment. *Journal of Psychosocial Oncology 4*(1/2), 19-31.

Scarce, M. (1999). The boys who bareback: Ride on the wild side, *POZ (The Journal for the HIV-Positive Community),* A54.

Shadish, W.R. and Montgomery, L.M. (1993). Effects of family and marital and marital psychotherapy: A meta-analysis. *Journal of Consulting and Clinical Psychology 61*(6), 992-1002.

Shelby, R.D. (1992). *If a Partner Has AIDS: Guide to Clinical Intervention for Relationships in Crisis.* Binghamton, NY: The Haworth Press.

Shelby, R.D. (1995). *People with HIV and Those Who Help Them: Challenges, Integration, Intervention.* Binghamton, NY: The Haworth Press.

Sigerist, H.E. (1943). *Civilization and Disease.* Ithaca, NY: Cornell University Press.

Sonnenberg-Schwa, U., Jaeger, U., Reuter, H., and Hammel, G. (1993). HIV-discordant couples: Artificial insemination with processed sperm—Psychological and psychosocial implications. *International Conference* 9(1), 524.

Spexiele, B.A. (1997). Couples, sexual intimacy, and multiple sclerosis. *Journal of Family Psychotherapy* 8(1), 133-152.

Sprenkle, D., Blow, A.A., and Dickey, M.H. (1999). Common factors and other non-technique variables in marriage and family therapy. In M. Hubble, B. Duncan, and C. Miller (Eds.), *The Heart and Soul of Change* (pp. 329-359). Washington, DC: APA Press.

St. Lawrence, J.S., Husfeldt, B.A., Kelly, J., Hoos, H.V., and Smith, S. (1990). The stigma of AIDS: Fear and diagnosis and prejudice towards gay men. *Journal of Homosexuality 19,* 85-101.

Strug, D., Grube, B., and Beckerman, N.L. (2002). Challenges and changing roles in HIV/AIDS Social Work: Implications for training and education. *Social Work in Health Care 35*(4), 1-19.

Stuart, R.B. (1969). Operant-interpersonal treatment for marital discord. *Journal of Consulting and Clinical Psychology 33,* 675-682.

Stulberg, I. and Buckingham, S. (1988). Parallel issues for AIDS patients, families, and others. *Social Casework: The Journal of Contemporary Social Work 69,* 145-159.

Swanstrom, R. and Erona, A. (2000). HIV type 1 protease inhibitors: Therapeutic successes and failures, suppression and resistance. *Pharmacological Therapy 86*(2), 145-170.

Tangenberg, K. (2003). Gender, geography, culture, and health: Emerging interdisciplinary approaches to global HIV/AIDS services. *Journal of Social Work Research and Evaluation 4*(1), 37-48.

Van der Straten, A., Vernon, K., Knight, K., Gomez, C., and Padian, N. (1998). Managing HIV among serodiscordant heterosexual couples: Serostatus, stigma, and sex. *AIDS Care 10*(5), 533-548.

VanDevanter, N., Clearly, P.D., and Moore, J. (1998). Reproductive behavior in HIV-discordant heterosexual couples: Implications for counseling. *AIDS Patient Care and STDs 12*(1), 43-49.

VanDevanter, N., Thacker, A.S., Bass, G., and Arnold, M. (1999). Heterosexual couples confronting the challenges of HIV infection. *AIDS Care 11,* 181-193.

Vittinghoff, E., Sheer, S., O'Malley, P., Colfax, G., Holmberg, S.D., and Buchbinder, S.P. (1999). Combination antiretroviral therapy and recent declines in AIDS incidence and mortality. *Journal of Infectious Disease 179*(4), 717-720.

VonBertalanffy, L. (1968). *General Systems Theory.* New York: George Brazilian.

Walker, G. (1991). *In the Midst of Winter: Systemic Therapy with Families, Couples and Individuals with AIDS infection.* New York: W.W. Norton and Company.

Weitz, R. (1989). Uncertainty and the lives of persons with AIDS. *Journal of Health and Social Behavior 30*(1), 18-29.

Wile, D.B. (1995). The ego-analytic approach to couple therapy. In N.S. Jacobsen and A.S. Gurman (Eds.), *Clinical Handbook of Couple Therapy* (pp. 91-120). New York: The Guilford Press.

Williams-Saporito, J. (1998). The effects of time-limited support group for married, heterosexual, serodiscordant couples. Third Annual HIV and Diversity Conference at Wurzweiler School of Social Work, November 19.

Winiarski, M. (1991). *AIDS-Related Psychotherapy.* New York: Pergamon Press.

Yep, G.A., Lovaas, K.E., and Pagonis, A.V. (2002). The case of "riding bareback": Sexual practices and the paradoxes of identity in the era of AIDS. *Journal of Homosexuality 42*(4), 1-14.

Index

Page numbers followed by the letter "t" indicate tables.

Order a copy of this book with this form or online at:

http://www.haworthpress.com/store/product.asp?sku=5327

COUPLES OF MIXED HIV STATUS
Clinical Issues and Interventions

_____in hardbound at $34.95 (ISBN: 0-7890-1851-9)

_____in softbound at $22.95 (ISBN: 0-7890-1852-7)

Or order online and use special offer code HEC25 in the shopping cart.

COST OF BOOKS_____

☐ **BILL ME LATER:** (Bill-me option is good on US/Canada/Mexico orders only; not good to jobbers, wholesalers, or subscription agencies.)

☐ Check here if billing address is different from shipping address and attach purchase order and billing address information.

POSTAGE & HANDLING_____
(US: $4.00 for first book & $1.50 for each additional book)
(Outside US: $5.00 for first book & $2.00 for each additional book)

Signature_____

SUBTOTAL_____

☐ **PAYMENT ENCLOSED: $**_____

IN CANADA: ADD 7% GST_____

☐ **PLEASE CHARGE TO MY CREDIT CARD.**

STATE TAX_____
(NJ, NY, OH, MN, CA, IL, IN, PA, & SD residents, add appropriate local sales tax)

☐ Visa ☐ MasterCard ☐ AmEx ☐ Discover
☐ Diner's Club ☐ Eurocard ☐ JCB

Account #_____

FINAL TOTAL_____
(If paying in Canadian funds, convert using the current exchange rate, UNESCO coupons welcome)

Exp. Date_____

Signature_____

Prices in US dollars and subject to change without notice.

NAME_____

INSTITUTION_____

ADDRESS_____

CITY_____

STATE/ZIP_____

COUNTRY_____ COUNTY (NY residents only)_____

TEL_____ FAX_____

E-MAIL_____

May we use your e-mail address for confirmations and other types of information? ☐ Yes ☐ No
We appreciate receiving your e-mail address and fax number. Haworth would like to e-mail or fax special discount offers to you, as a preferred customer. **We will never share, rent, or exchange your e-mail address or fax number.** We regard such actions as an invasion of your privacy.

Order From Your Local Bookstore or Directly From

The Haworth Press, Inc.

10 Alice Street, Binghamton, New York 13904-1580 • USA
TELEPHONE: 1-800-HAWORTH (1-800-429-6784) / Outside US/Canada: (607) 722-5857
FAX: 1-800-895-0582 / Outside US/Canada: (607) 771-0012
E-mail to: orders@haworthpress.com

For orders outside US and Canada, you may wish to order through your local
sales representative, distributor, or bookseller.
For information, see http://haworthpress.com/distributors

(Discounts are available for individual orders in US and Canada only, not booksellers/distributors.)

PLEASE PHOTOCOPY THIS FORM FOR YOUR PERSONAL USE.

http://www.HaworthPress.com

BOF04